Warwickshire County Council

THE NATURAL MENOPAUSE PLAN

How to overcome the symptons
with diet, supplements, exercise
and more than 90 recipes

MARYON STEWART

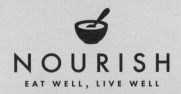

NOURISH

EAT WELL, LIVE WELL

THE NATURAL MENOPAUSE PLAN
MARYON STEWART

To Rosa, Sue and Phoebe – my mother, sister and daughter –
with gratitude for your constant support and inspiration

First published in the UK and USA in 2011 by
Duncan Baird Publishers Ltd

This edition published in the UK and USA in 2017 by
Nourish, an imprint of Watkins Media Limited
19 Cecil Court
London WC2N 4EZ

enquiries@nourishbooks.com

Managing Editor: Grace Cheetham
Editor: Kesta Desmond
Design: Georgina Hewitt & Karen Smith
Commissioned photography: William Lingwood
Food Stylist: Lucy McKelvie
Prop Stylist: Wei Tang

A CIP record for this book is available from the British Library

ISBN: 978 1 84899 330 3

10 9 8 7 6 5 4 3 2 1

Typeset in Brandon Grotesque and MrsEaves
Colour reproduction by XY Digital
Printed in China

Publisher's note
While every care has been taken in compiling the recipes for this
book, Watkins Media Limited, or any other persons who have been
involved in working on this publication, cannot accept responsibility
for any errors or omissions, inadvertent or not, that may be found
in the recipes or text, nor for any problems that may arise as a
result of preparing one of these recipes. If you are pregnant or
breastfeeding or have any special dietary requirements or medical
conditions, it is advisable to consult a medical professional before
following any of the recipes contained in this book.

Notes on the recipes
Unless otherwise stated:
Use medium (US large) organic or free-range eggs
Use fresh herbs, spices and chillies
Use granulated sugar (Americans can use ordinary granulated sugar
when caster sugar is specified)
Do not mix metric, imperial and US cup measurements:
1 tsp = 5ml 1 tbsp = 15ml 1 cup = 240ml

nourishbooks.com

CONTENTS

INTRODUCTION

You may be nearing the menopause, you may have already reached it, or you may even be coming out the other end and wondering how to protect your heart, bones and memory in the long term. You probably don't know which way to turn, as there is so much conflicting advice out there. Should you just put up with the symptoms? Should you go on hormone replacement therapy (HRT) although you don't particularly want to? Or should you try some of the many natural and herbal supplements available and, if so, which ones? And what if you're already taking HRT – should you carry on or should you come off because of the long-term implications?

You have every reason to be confused. The newspapers and media, not to mention doctors and nurses, are full of advice on the best ways to approach this important stage in your life, yet they don't always agree with each other and many of the options offered are not even vaguely scientifically based.

The most popular treatment for menopausal symptoms over the past 20 years has been HRT. However, several major international HRT studies have now been aborted owing to the increased risk of serious medical conditions for participants, such as heart disease, stroke, thrombosis, breast cancer and ovarian cancer. Understandably, many women are now looking for an alternative treatment to HRT.

The natural way of managing your menopause

The Natural Menopause Plan is a scientifically based, natural, proven alternative to hormone replacement therapy. Over the past 20 years, we at the Natural Health Advisory Service (NHAS) have pioneered this simple, workable and enjoyable plan to help alleviate your symptoms during the years leading up to your last period and beyond. The plan is based on sound research and extensive clinical practice, and the success rate, within a matter of months, astounds most of our patients and is a constant source of satisfaction for our dedicated team of health professionals.

Many years of working with women at the NHAS (and carrying out research projects to measure levels of nutrients in women at different life stages) has led me to realize that falling levels of estrogen are not the only trigger of menopausal symptoms. There are other things to blame.

Factors such as diet and lifestyle play a part. Pregnancy, breastfeeding and physical and mental stress also take their toll on our wellbeing. Levels of some nutrients drop naturally as we age. Taking all this into account, it's not surprising that by the time many women reach the menopause, they are firing on two cylinders instead of four. As a result, if they are not in a good nutritional or physiological state, their menopausal symptoms and long-term health prospects are likely to be more severe.

Once we realize that menopausal symptoms are not all to do with falling levels of estrogen, and that other physical and mental factors are involved, it follows that any successful programme must address all three areas. So it's no coincidence that our Natural Menopause Plan encompasses all these factors with consistently fantastic results. A recent survey showed that more than 91 percent of women who followed our plan felt that their estrogen withdrawal symptoms were under control within five months, and their physical and mental symptoms significantly improved too.

Tailoring the plan to your needs

The trick is to find the right approach for you, one which allows you to control your symptoms, rather than allowing them to control you. This is where the Natural Menopause Plan can really help you. In Part 1, I explain how you can adapt your diet and lifestyle to address your menopausal symptoms and to ensure the long-term health of your heart, bones and other body systems. As you read Part 1, make a note of the specific supplements, foods, nutrients, therapies and lifestyle changes that address your particular symptoms and health issues. Part 2 of the book is devoted to a wide selection of delicious recipes – these are specifically designed to help you move toward a diet rich in phytoestrogens.

As you start following the Natural Menopause Plan diet, try using my phyto-rich menu plans (see page 146). I've also included comprehensive food charts (see page 150), so if you need to top up your levels of a particular vitamin, mineral or essential fatty acid, you'll know exactly what to eat. I hope that within weeks of beginning the Natural Menopause Plan, you'll notice your symptoms abating and a new level of vitality emerging. Start by turning the page to read some inspiring stories from women who have already tried the plan.

YOUR STORIES

I was taken by surprise by my menopausal symptoms and I admit it was somewhat of a shock to have reached that stage in my life. I found myself suddenly suffering appalling anxiety, I became easily wound up about very small things and was left feeling desperately tired as a result of my sleep being disrupted by the night sweats. When I had a hot flush while I was working, I couldn't concentrate on what my director was saying, which I found both disconcerting and embarrassing. Maryon was recommended by a friend in whom I confided and thankfully it was only three or four weeks after seeing her that I started feeling better. I cut out caffeine and used decaffeinated drinks and cut back on alcohol as every time I had a glass of wine I began flushing. I used soy milk and yogurt instead of dairy and that was a huge help, too. Plus I took the supplements Fema 45+, Promensil and high-strength fish oils, and made sure I did regular exercise. I hurt my back shortly after starting Maryon's programme, so I had some acupuncture which definitely helped as well. I feel 500 percent better now. I'm more energetic, I haven't got any of the symptoms and I feel like a completely different person, which is truly wonderful.

CHERIE LUNGHI, ACTRESS

I had been on HRT following a hysterectomy. When I looked in the mirror, I saw a stranger. My eyes looked blank and listless, my skin colour had changed and it appeared thinner. I felt like I wanted to go to bed, but I was afraid to because I knew I would wake up and not be able to get back to sleep again. I had gained 13kg (28lb) on HRT and felt awful about myself. It felt as if I had a burning fire in my vagina, and I was moody and listless. I had low blood pressure and often felt dizzy. I was constantly worried about everything and nothing.

I read about the NHAS in a magazine. I immediately called them to arrange a telephone consultation. I was given a series of recommendations to follow and went about implementing them. My first follow-up appointment was six weeks later, by which time all my severe symptoms were mild. I had so much energy, I couldn't believe the difference. In another four weeks, I could only describe myself as a different person. Maryon weaned me off the HRT, I lost weight, my vagina feels normal and my libido is back. Everyone says how great I look and I certainly feel it.

LYNN CARR, SPECIAL NEEDS TEACHER

My worst symptoms were the regular and intense hot flushes resulting in an overwhelming sense of lethargy. It turned me into a stranger and even my family said I had such a poor quality of life that it needed to be addressed. I was delighted to find Maryon Stewart's book and felt comforted to discover that there was a solution to my troubles. I had an initial consultation with her and she gave me a series of recommendations, which included making dietary changes, taking supplements, exercising and relaxation. I included soy and roasted flaxseeds in my diet, which made a difference to my symptoms. Even though I'm not really a "pill person", I took Promensil and found that the benefits far outweighed any misgivings I had. Within a month, I noticed the intensity of my symptoms had reduced. Over the next month, the flushes almost completely disappeared and I got my energy back. I went from having no real quality of life to feeling absolutely excellent!

MERLE SHAPIRO, JEWELLERY DESIGNER

My hot flushes came on slowly, but before very long they just escalated. I was awake four or five times during each night and I couldn't get back to sleep after I'd had a night sweat. It was impossible to cuddle up with my husband. I had to push him away, as physical contact made the flushes worse. The lack of sleep made it very difficult to function during the day and to cope with my job as a nurse. I became moody and got irritable with clients. I got so desperate that I asked my doctor to prescribe HRT, but he didn't want me to go on it and suggested I just go it alone. I didn't really know where to start at first. I tried taking black cohosh, but then I read that it may cause liver damage. I changed my diet by cutting out caffeine, alcohol and spicy food, all of which seemed to make the symptoms worse. Then I started taking Promensil. After about two months, I noticed big changes. The hot flushes and night sweats reduced dramatically and I started sleeping through the night. I could cuddle up to my husband again and felt so much better once I was sleeping properly. I am now a much happier person. My family has noticed a big difference in my attitude and my children have commented that I'm not moody and snappy any more. I feel much more like my old self and happy to be managing my menopause naturally.

DONNA LOTHIAN, NURSE PRACTITIONER

I approached the NHAS for help with my headaches and fatigue, which had become worse since taking HRT. I changed my diet as instructed, including foods that contained naturally occurring estrogen and phytoestrogen-rich supplements, and began doing regular exercise and relaxation. After a few weeks, I had so much more energy. My friends also commented on how clear my skin looked. I'd been treated for high blood pressure and both my consultant and my doctor were amazed to find that, since embarking on the NHAS programme, my blood pressure had returned to the normal range and my cholesterol level had reduced from 5.9 to 5.4.

JEAN CUNNINGHAM, RETIRED CIVIL SERVANT

I was put on HRT at the age of 41 as I was suffering with anxiety and depression. Both my sister and my mother had an early menopause and, sure enough, when I went to my doctor I discovered that my FSH was elevated, which meant I was perimenopausal. I began taking the HRT as directed, but my migraines became intolerable. I was given medication for them, which seemed to work for a while but became less effective over time. I was also experiencing anxiety attacks and felt depressed and tired for much of the time. It wasn't helped by the fact that I had lost my mum and my mother-in-law in the space of a couple of years. I used to get very bloated and constipated and my libido was almost non-existent to the point where sex was off the menu.

I saw Maryon in her clinic and got started on her recommendations. Within four weeks, I noticed my migraines were completely gone. I used to get at least two a month for years, and that got even worse once I began taking the HRT.

Maryon weaned me off the HRT over a couple of months and I took supplements, including Femenessence, to control my hot flushes and night sweats. Within three months I was laughing and joking with my kids again. I felt like I'd got my sparkle back. Within another few months I felt even better. My relationships with my children and my husband were entirely different and I wanted to do things with them instead of sitting around feeling exhausted. Life didn't feel like a drudge any more and, as a bonus, my libido returned. Recently I was invited to apply for a job for which there were 60 applicants. Amazingly I got it. I know that I wouldn't even have felt up to applying before. I feel so much better than I did on HRT, in fact, I've never felt better.

JANICE GILLETT, ADMINISTRATOR IN ADULT LEARNING

I went through an early menopause in my early 40s. I had a bone density scan and was shocked to discover a seven percent loss of bone mass in one year. I was advised to take long-term medication, but after reading about Maryon Stewart's natural alternatives, I decided to give myself a year trying natural solutions before accepting the drugs as inevitable.

I went and saw Maryon, who helped me refine my programme. This involved making significant dietary changes, taking nutritional supplements and doing daily weight-bearing exercises. A year later, my follow-up bone density scan showed almost no further bone loss and the advice this time was "keep taking the tablets". I'm hoping next year's scan will show I have made some new bone. I'm certainly feeling well and much fitter as a result of my new regime.

JOANNE SIMMS, MOTHER OF TWO

My menopausal symptoms began shortly after a partial hysterectomy when I was 45. I had night sweats that severely disrupted my sleep, leaving me exhausted. I also had a high cholesterol level.

I didn't want to take HRT and preferred to make changes to my diet in order to control my symptoms. Reducing caffeine helped and I ate roasted flaxseeds daily. Within a few months my flushes diminished and my quality and quantity of sleep improved. My cholesterol levels also returned to normal for the first time in three years. In addition, I noticed that my hair became healthier looking, my skin got back its old glow and I had much more energy.

LAURIE CAMPBELL, ADMINISTRATOR

I had horrendous hot flushes, night and day, which ruined my last term as a full-time lecturer and wrecked my life. I'm not exaggerating! During the night, I had up to 12 hot flushes and sweats and probably twice this during the day. Sweat would literally run down my face. I felt completely debilitated and low in confidence, since I never knew when a flush or sweat would strike. Within a week of starting the NHAS programme, my energy levels and sense of wellbeing returned. Within a few months of following the recommended diet, including soy products, taking the recommended supplements and doing my exercise and relaxation, the flushes were non-existent. I was miraculously back to my old self again, and totally cool and calm!

ANN HIGGINS, LECTURER

Like many things in life, menopause has its pros and cons and can bring a complex mix of emotions. While most women are delighted that they no longer have a monthly period, many of the other signs and symptoms of menopause are not so welcome. Fortunately, the Natural Menopause Plan, which is based on the successful programme we've been running at the Natural Health Advisory Service (NHAS) for more than 20 years, provides a simple, workable and enjoyable way to alleviate all your symptoms and restore a sense of vitality and self-esteem.

In Part 1, I explain what's going on in your body during the perimenopause, what the menopause is, why it happens and what sort of symptoms – physical and emotional – you may experience. I put hormone replacement therapy (HRT) into perspective and explain alternative natural ways to manage your symptoms. I also explain how you can protect your long-term health. Most importantly, I introduce the principles of my Natural Menopause Plan: a phytoestrogen-rich diet; scientifically proven supplements; and complementary therapies that enhance your health. One thing I've noticed in our patients is that after following the Natural Menopause Plan they regain their zest for life, their physical shape and self-esteem and often end up feeling better than they can ever remember.

As you start implementing the recommended changes in Part 1, keep a diet diary and complete a daily symptom chart. Do this for the first three to four months to help you monitor your progress. Follow the plan for at least four to six months to gain optimum benefit.

PART 1
Understanding the Menopause

WHAT'S HAPPENING TO ME?

One night, out of the blue, you find yourself waking up in a hot sweat. You throw off the covers, even though the room temperature is freezing. At first, this only happens occasionally. But as time goes on, it becomes a nightly occurrence, disrupting your sleep and leaving you worn out the next day.

And your days aren't that much better. Increasingly, you start feeling waves of heat rising through your body, often when you get hot, or in moments of stress, such as when you're sitting in a traffic jam, in a meeting or on a crowded train. Your periods become erratic and your moods are like those of a teenager. What on earth is going on? You're not ill, nor are you going mad. This is the run-up to your menopause.

Menopause literally means the last day of your last period, although most of us use the word pretty loosely to describe the various symptoms that we experience in the years before and after this event. It can happen any time between the ages of 45 and 55, with 51 being the average. The general consensus is that you have passed your menopause when you have stopped menstruating for one year, which is why the menopause can only be accurately dated in hindsight.

WHY DOES THE MENOPAUSE HAPPEN?

At birth, your ovaries contain thousands of follicles, or egg sacs, in which egg cells ripen and develop. At puberty, your ovaries start to release an egg each month under the influence of two chemical messengers, or hormones, produced by the pituitary gland in the brain. These two hormones, follicle-stimulating hormone (FSH) and luteinizing hormone (LH), in turn trigger your ovaries to produce two more hormones, estrogen and progesterone, which are responsible for preparing the lining of your womb for pregnancy. If an egg is not fertilized, estrogen and progesterone levels decline and the egg, together with the build-up of womb lining, is shed in the form of a period.

As you go through your 40s, the supply of eggs you were born with starts to run out and your ovaries stop releasing an egg each month. This means you no longer produce so much progesterone and estrogen, and your hormone levels fluctuate from one month to the next. Eventually, your ovaries run out of eggs altogether, progesterone production ceases and estrogen levels fall. Estrogen is required for many bodily functions – not just for reproduction – including strong bones, a sharp mind and a healthy heart, so it is inevitable that you will feel the effects of decreasing estrogen.

WHAT IS THE PERIMENOPAUSE?

Your body goes through a series of changes leading up to the menopause. These are known collectively as the "perimenopause" ("peri" meaning "around"). The first sign that things are on the move is usually a change in the pattern of your periods. They may become irregular, longer or shorter, as well as heavier or, in some cases, lighter. Many of us are unprepared for the perimenopause. It can simply bring a degree of unpredictability into your life, since you never know when your period will arrive. If you are less fortunate, you can experience a worsening of PMS symptoms (see page 17), as well as mood swings and more "black" days than you dare to count. Other symptoms include:

- ◆ hot flushes
- ◆ night sweats
- ◆ mood swings
- ◆ loss of libido
- ◆ loss of energy
- ◆ sleepless nights
- ◆ not being able to concentrate

WHAT CAUSES PREMATURE MENOPAUSE?

In about one percent of women the menopause happens before the age of 40. This is known as premature menopause or premature ovarian failure (POF). The symptoms are the same as those of a natural menopause. You are more likely to have a premature menopause if you fall into any of these categories.

· *You have your ovaries removed by surgery (oophorectomy), which sometimes happens during a hysterectomy if your ovaries are abnormal; or to prevent the spread of endometriosis or ovarian or endometrial cancer.*

· *You have radiotherapy or chemotherapy for the treatment of leukemia or cancer.*

· *You have a family history (hereditary cause) of premature menopause, or a chromosomal defect.*

· *You smoke. (Research shows that smoking is strongly linked with premature menopause. Heavy smokers can reach the menopause up to two years earlier than non-smokers.)*

· *You had your last child before you were 28.*

· *You have never had children.*

· *You are short or underweight.*

· *Your diet is nutritionally poor.*

RECOGNIZING MENOPAUSAL SIGNS

If your periods start to become erratic, or you haven't had a period for several months, this could be the beginning of your menopause. It's useful to be aware of menopausal changes because then you can take prompt action to preserve your short- and long-term health.

The quickest way to discover whether you're menopausal is to ask your doctor to do a test, or to do one yourself at home. The test examines levels of follicle-stimulating hormone (FSH) in your urine. As you go into the menopause, levels of FSH rise dramatically and can remain high for two years, or until your brain gets the message that your ovaries are no longer producing estrogen. At this point, FSH drops back to premenopausal levels. Because FSH levels fluctuate during the menstrual cycle, you'll need to do a home test twice (with a week between tests). If FSH levels are high only on one of the tests, it's unlikely that you're menopausal, but if both tests show a high reading, this confirms your menopausal status.

TYPES OF SYMPTOMS

Your symptoms can alert you to the fact that you are menopausal. Symptoms can be divided into three main groups: estrogen withdrawal symptoms; other physical symptoms; and mental/emotional symptoms.

ESTROGEN WITHDRAWAL SYMPTOMS

- Hot flushes
- Night sweats
- Urinary symptoms
- Loss of libido
- Vaginal dryness
- Difficulties with intercourse

OTHER PHYSICAL SYMPTOMS

- Aches and pains
- Migraines and headaches
- Fatigue
- Constipation
- Irritable bowel syndrome

MENTAL/EMOTIONAL SYMPTOMS

- Anxiety and panic attacks
- Irritability
- Mood swings
- Depression
- Confusion and/ or memory loss

HOW DOES A HISTORY OF PMS AFFECT MENOPAUSE?

Premenstrual syndrome (PMS) refers to the physical and mental symptoms that can occur just before the arrival of a period, and which then diminish or disappear shortly afterwards. For some women, PMS becomes even worse around the time of the menopause. A study we carried out at the Natural Health Advisory Service (NHAS) looked at the relationship between previous PMS symptoms and current menopausal symptoms. Mental symptoms did seem to show some kind of continuity from PMS to the menopause, with a small connection in relation to symptoms such as anxiety, depression, confusion and insomnia.

However, there was little or no link with physical symptoms, such as hot flushes and night sweats, suggesting that symptoms mainly due to estrogen withdrawal are not greatly influenced by a history of PMS. In our experience, diet and lifestyle seem to make a big difference to many women's PMS symptoms, which is good news if you are going through similar mood changes at the time of the menopause.

WHAT CAUSES MENOPAUSAL SYMPTOMS?

Fluctuating hormone levels are a key trigger of menopausal symptoms, but they're not solely responsible. The many surveys that we have carried out at the NHAS suggest that dietary and lifestyle factors at this time of life also play a significant part in determining the severity of symptoms. Pregnancy and breastfeeding, as well as nutritional imbalances that may have developed over many years as a result of dieting, poor eating habits or malabsorption, can often take their toll, leaving many of us in a nutritionally depleted state as we enter the menopausal years.

The menopause also tends to hit most of us at a psychological turning point, when natural fears about ageing and what the future may hold start weighing on our minds. In your mid-to-late forties and early fifties, you can find yourself overloaded with other problems, such as the ups and downs of life with teenage children, caring for elderly relatives, changes in your relationship (if you have one) or perhaps doing a job outside the home for the first time in years. If, on top of all this, you have the menopause to deal with, it's not surprising if you feel below par!

Despite the changes you may be experiencing, it's important to keep things in perspective. The menopause needn't be the end of life as you knew it, but rather the beginning of a new phase that can be just as rewarding. If you take into account all the causes of your symptoms, there's much you can do to make this transition as smooth as possible.

HRT IN FOCUS

Until fairly recently, hormone replacement therapy (HRT) was considered a major breakthrough in the treatment of the menopause – and many doctors thought of it as a treatment for life. It seemed to provide the perfect answer to short-term discomforts, such as hot flushes, night sweats, mood swings and a dry vagina. It was also seen as a protector against longer-term risks, such as heart disease and osteoporosis. It seemed there wasn't a symptom it couldn't help...

Today, following the results of a number of international studies, a different story is beginning to emerge. It now seems, rather than being a cure-all, HRT can increase the risk of breast cancer and may not protect the heart. As a result, the medical fraternity has had to think again.

It has now been recommended that HRT should be prescribed only in the lowest dose needed to bring short-term symptoms under control, and for the shortest possible time – if at all. Doctors are advised to review women taking HRT at least annually. If symptoms persist, doctors should re-prescribe HRT only for a maximum of five years, rather than a lifetime. Once symptoms have been alleviated, women should be weaned off HRT and encouraged to use an alternative approach.

If you still want to try HRT, read the list on page 19 to check that you don't have any health issues that would prevent you taking it. And be aware that HRT can aggravate migraines, multiple sclerosis, epilepsy, diabetes, high blood pressure (occasionally), gallstones and premenstrual syndrome (PMS). Plus there are common initial side-effects that include: breast tenderness and enlargement; PMS symptoms, such as mood swings; nausea and vomiting; possible weight gain; breakthrough vaginal bleeding mid-cycle; leg cramps; enlargement of pre-existing uterine fibroids; intolerance of contact lenses; patchy increase in skin pigmentation; hair loss from the scalp; and an increase in body or facial hair.

THE ALTERNATIVE TO HRT

After 20 years of helping women through their health problems at the Natural Health Advisory Service, I can put my hand on my heart and say with certainty that an effective, scientifically based, natural alternative to HRT is available. My Natural Menopause Plan will help you to overcome menopausal symptoms, and to protect yourself against heart disease and osteoporosis in the longer term. The Natural Menopause Plan is based on a phytoestrogen-rich diet and a selection of recommended supplements, plus moderate exercise and relaxation. I'll explain all the principles in the pages that follow. If you are currently taking HRT and wish to stop, you should wean yourself off

HOW TO WEAN YOURSELF OFF HRT

Before you attempt to come off HRT, you need to be established on the Natural Menopause Plan. So start to wean yourself off HRT only after four to six weeks of your new eating and supplement routine. Then you should reduce HRT gradually (stopping suddenly can lead to fairly severe withdrawal symptoms). If you're on a high-dose HRT pill or patch, ask your doctor to prescribe a lower dose for a month or two before coming off HRT.

Then halve your dose for approximately one month as follows:
• *If you're taking pills, break them in half or take one every second day.*
• *If you use patches, cut them in half or use one every second day.*
• *If you use a nasal spray, use it less or on alternate days.*

When you decide the time is right, choose a day on which to stop taking HRT altogether. If you experience mild flushes during the next couple of months, simply increase the amount of isoflavones (see page 26) you eat on a daily basis. And also increase your intake of red clover (see page 32) in the short term.

gradually (see box on page 19). At the NHAS we conducted two studies on women coming off HRT. Both studies showed that over 91 percent of the women were weaned off HRT successfully, without any side-effects or symptoms, within five months.

WHEN YOU SHOULD AVOID HRT

You should not take HRT if any of the following apply to you:
• *A family history of breast or ovarian cancer.*
• *Abnormal vaginal bleeding that has not yet been diagnosed.*
• *Endometriosis (where the womb lining grows, and subsequently bleeds, outside the womb).*
• *Severe cardiac, liver or kidney disease.*
• *An impending operation within the next six weeks (an operation can increase the risk of thrombosis).*
• *Uterine fibroids (HRT can cause heavier bleeding).*
• *Diabetes (HRT can change blood sugar levels).*
• *Breast cysts or pain.*
• *A personal or strong family history of thrombosis (blood clots), especially if you are a smoker.*

NATURAL SYMPTOM RELIEF

We all respond differently to the menopause. Some women sail through it and wonder what all the fuss is about. But for many others, the hormonal swings bring about body changes and unwanted symptoms that can disrupt their lives and result in misery. The good news is that all these symptoms can be overcome with simple diet and lifestyle adjustments. The only side-effect will be that you feel more like your old self or, in many cases, a whole lot better!

HOT FLUSHES AND NIGHT SWEATS

No-one knows for sure what causes hot flushes, but it's thought that a lack of estrogen may affect the action of the hypothalamus, the region of the brain that controls body temperature. More than 80 percent of women are thought to be affected at some point. Flushes can often start long before you stop menstruating and can continue for several years afterwards.

The frequency, duration and intensity of hot flushes vary from one woman to another. You may get several a day, or be plagued constantly day and night. They can last from a few seconds to around five minutes, with four minutes being the average. As well as the sudden rush of heat, you may experience a racing heart, dizziness, anxiety and irritability.

Night sweats are severe hot flushes. You can wake up simply drenched in sweat. You may even have to change your night clothes and your sheets. If you repeatedly wake up this way, night after night, fatigue and exhaustion will soon set in. Physical contact with your partner can also trigger a flush, which may mean you're less keen on physical intimacy – this in turn can lead to relationship problems if your partner starts to feel rejected.

HELP YOURSELF

- *Don't be embarrassed by a flush. The moment you feel one coming on, stop what you're doing. Take several slow, deep breaths and try to relax. This helps to reduce the severity of the attack.*
- *If possible, drink a glass of cold water and sit still until the flush passes.*
- *Wear layers of thin clothes that you can easily strip off when you feel yourself getting hot. Clothes made of natural fibres, such as cotton, help your skin to breathe.*
- *Keep your bedroom cool at night and keep a fan, wet wipes and a cold drink by your bed. Use cotton sheets and pillowcases, and wear cotton night clothes.*
- *Eat small, regular meals. The heat generated by the process of digesting a large meal can sometimes bring on a flush.*

- *Cut down on alcohol, caffeine, hot drinks and spicy foods, as these can all bring on flushes.*
- *Exercise regularly (see page 50).*
- *Quit smoking. Research shows that it increases the risk of flushing.*
- *Include plenty of polyunsaturated fats and isoflavones (see pages 26–7) in your diet. Research shows that about 100mg of isoflavones a day can control severe hot flushes. This should be consumed through both food and supplements. A regular intake of isoflavones helps keep blood estrogen levels elevated. As a rough guide, there are approximately 20mg of isoflavones in a 250ml/9fl oz glass of soy milk, 10mg in a 125g/4½oz/½ cup portion of soy yogurt or dessert, 25mg in 100g/3½oz of tofu and 7mg in a tablespoon of organic golden flaxseeds. Research confirms it's best to consume these foods in small quantities throughout the day, rather than in a single sitting.*
- *Try taking scientifically based supplements (see page 32).*

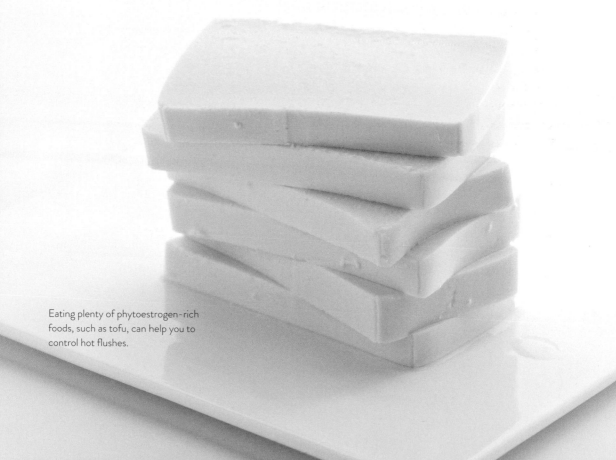

Eating plenty of phytoestrogen-rich foods, such as tofu, can help you to control hot flushes.

SEXUAL PROBLEMS

A lack of estrogen causes the vaginal lining to become thin and dry. There is also a decrease in vaginal muscle tone and blood supply to the urogenital area around the time of the menopause. The result is that sex becomes uncomfortable and, in some cases, painful. The good news is that this is reversible through diet and specialist supplements.

HELP YOURSELF

• *Phytoestrogen creams, such as Arkopharma Phyto Soya Vaginal Gel help to alleviate vaginal dryness and discomfort. Use the gel twice a week (clinical trials show it can help to rehydrate and restore the elasticity of vaginal tissues within three weeks). Use Yes organic gel on the other nights.*

• *Omega-7 capsules also help to ease vaginal dryness. Derived from sea buckthorn, a berry bush naturally found in Asia and Europe, omega 7 helps to maintain the health and integrity of the mucous membranes in the vagina. It has been used in traditional Asian medicine for more than 1,000 years. For women experiencing severe vaginal dryness or bleeding during sex, I recommend two capsules of PharmaNord's Omega-7 in the morning and two in the evening. You'll be delighted with the results.*

• *Don't stop having sex. Regular sex can help increase vaginal lubrication. If it takes longer to become aroused than it used to, ensure you and your partner enjoy a slow build-up to sex with plenty of foreplay.*

• *Pelvic floor exercises help to keep your vagina healthy and strengthen pelvic muscles. This in turn makes sex more pleasurable and helps to prevent urinary incontinence, which can become common in midlife. Locate the appropriate muscles by stopping a flow of urine mid-stream. Once you know where the muscles are, contract them 10–15 times a day using the following technique. With your legs slightly apart, draw your buttocks in. At the same time, draw your vagina inward and upward. Squeeze and hold for a few seconds.*

• *Take Promensil supplements (see page 32). Research shows they help to alleviate vaginal dryness.*

• *Read my guidelines about revving up your sex drive in the long term (see page 56).*

HEADACHES

Headaches and migraines are common during the menopause and can be the result of changing body temperature, tiredness due to hot flushes, sleeplessness, or general stress and anxiety. Migraines can be affected by estrogen levels; you may find that they get better or worse during the menopause.

HELP YOURSELF

• *Try relaxation techniques (see page 40).*

• *Regular exercise is essential (see page 50).*

- *Complementary therapies, such as massage and acupuncture, can help to ease the pain.*
- *Eat an oatcake before you go to bed to help keep blood sugar levels balanced. If your blood sugar drops during the night, you may wake up with a morning headache.*

EMOTIONAL SYMPTOMS

Depression, irritability, mood swings and anxiety are common menopausal symptoms and are probably caused by the hormonal and physical changes you are going through. It's important to realize that these feelings will pass, although it may take some time.

HELP YOURSELF

- *Don't bottle up your feelings or turn to alcohol, cigarettes or food for comfort. Instead, talk to a friend or a family member about how you're feeling.*
- *Follow the Natural Menopause Plan diet, which is rich in phytoestrogens (see page 26).*
- *Exercise regularly. Exercise has been shown to improve symptoms of depression and anxiety more effectively than psychotherapy. In a comparative study, after a 12-week aerobic programme, the women who exercised had fewer symptoms of depression and anxiety than women who had psychotherapy. At the follow-up session one year later, this was still the case.*
- *Try complementary therapies such as yoga (see page 41), and relaxation techniques, such as meditation.*

INSOMNIA

Sleepless nights can fast become the norm, so tackle them straight away. Usual causes include night sweats, anxiety or getting up to go to the toilet. Poor sleep can trigger other symptoms, such as depression and irritability, so if you start to sleep better, you may also notice an improvement in your mood.

HELP YOURSELF

- *Tackle the possible underlying causes of your insomnia, such as anxiety and night sweats.*
- *During the night, take the herb valerian (see page 38) to help you to get back to sleep until your night sweats are under control.*
- *Include some relaxation and exercise in your day.*
- *Avoid caffeine or alcohol before bedtime. Have a hot soy milk drink, camomile or valerian tea.*
- *Listen to soothing music to help you to relax and sleep soundly. Don't take worries to bed with you.*
- *Avoid watching, reading or listening to anything too stimulating in the evening.*
- *Fix a regular time to go to bed and to get up in the morning, so your body is accustomed to a pattern.*

DRY SKIN AND WRINKLES

Many women start to notice their skin becoming drier around the menopause. You may also notice an increase in wrinkles. This is due to the effect that lowered estrogen levels have on collagen, the skin's main structural protein that keeps skin firm by supporting and binding its connective tissue.

HELP YOURSELF

· *Moisturize frequently. I recommend Arkopharma Age Minimizing Cream. It is rich in phytoestrogen and has a three-fold anti-ageing action, boosting cell renewal, stimulating collagen synthesis and protecting against free radicals. Trials show it can help reduce the depth of wrinkles by up to 48% within four weeks.*
· *Protect your skin from sun damage. Apply sunscreen with an SPF of at least 15 on your face, neck and hands.*
· *Drink at least eight glasses of water daily to keep your skin hydrated.*
· *Regularly exfoliate your skin so that your moisturizer can penetrate more easily.*
· *Eat plenty of oily fish, such as salmon and sardines. These are rich in omega-3 fatty acids, which will help to keep your skin soft and smooth.*

ACHING JOINTS

Lack of estrogen and essential nutrients at the time of the menopause can result in creaking bones and aching joints, especially first thing in the morning.

HELP YOURSELF

· *Fish oils have been the subject of many clinical trials and are proven to help relieve joint pain. In particular, eicosapantaenoic acid (EPA) in fish oil has been found to help arthritis. The omega-3 fatty acids in EPA create anti-inflammatory prostaglandins that ease the inflammation and pain of swollen joints. Try to eat two to three servings of oily fish, such as salmon, mackerel, herring, sardines or pilchards each week.*
· *Take a high-strength fish-oil supplement that contains more than 80 percent of omega-3 fatty acids, of which at least 50 percent is EPA.*
· *Take a glucosamine sulphate and chondroitin supplement (see page 35). Evidence suggests that glucosamine and chondroitin can reduce inflammation and pain, and aid joint movement. Regenovex also helps to reduce joint pain and inflammation.*
· *Eat at least five portions of fruit and vegetables a day.*
· *Most days, exercise to the point of breathlessness for at least 30 minutes. In the morning, try to fit in some stretching exercises to get you going.*
· *Don't smoke, and try to limit alcohol consumption to no more than three alcoholic drinks a week.*

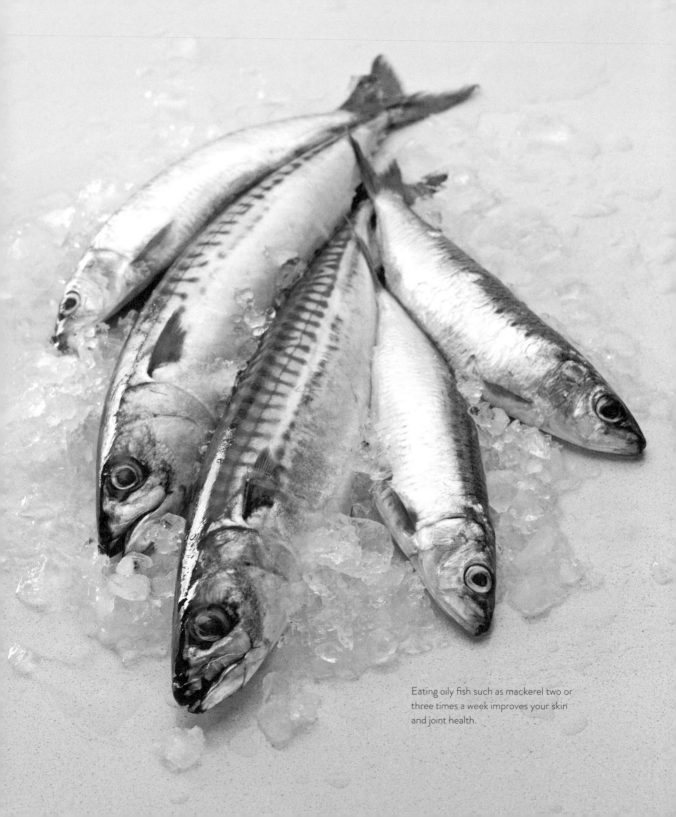

Eating oily fish such as mackerel two or three times a week improves your skin and joint health.

THE NATURAL MENOPAUSE PLAN DIET

The food we eat has a major impact on the range and severity of our menopausal symptoms. It's fascinating to note that Asian women have a very different experience of the menopause to Western women. They rarely experience hot flushes and night sweats and, until recently, the Japanese language didn't even include the term "hot flush". The key difference between the Western and Asian diets is the amount of plant estrogens – known as phytoestrogens – that are eaten.

A wealth of research in recent years has shown that a regular intake of phytoestrogens throughout the day can play a useful part in a menopause control programme in a similar way to HRT. In fact, although phytoestrogens are only about 1/1000th as potent as animal-based estrogen, they are fast becoming known as great hormone regulators owing to their balancing effects on estrogen levels. Here's how they work. When estrogen is in oversupply in the body, as can happen in women of reproductive age, phytoestrogens play musical chairs with estrogen, competing for the receptor sites in cells (receptors are structures found on the surfaces of cells that allow hormones and other chemicals into cells, rather like a key in a lock). Some of the phytoestrogens inevitably displace estrogen and, being so much weaker in effect, can help reduce the cancer-promoting effects of the hormone. On the other hand, as estrogen levels start to drop around the time of the menopause and beyond, phytoestrogens can give your levels a natural boost. Research shows that a diet rich in phytoestrogens combined with supplements and relaxation can alleviate menopausal symptoms,

GOOD SOURCES OF PHYTOESTROGENS

ISOFLAVONES

- soy milk
- soy beans
- tofu
- soy flour
- soy nuts
- beans and lentils
- chickpeas
- mung beans
- alfalfa
- red clover

LIGNANS

- flaxseeds
- sesame seeds
- sunflower seeds
- pumpkin seeds
- almonds
- green and yellow vegetables

improve cognitive function, restore memory and protect against heart disease. Phytoestrogens may also help to prevent osteoporosis. A study of 650 women aged between 19 and 86 found that postmenopausal women with the highest intake of dietary isoflavones had significantly higher bone mineral density in their spines and hips than those with the lowest intakes (after adjusting other factors such as age, height, weight, years since the menopause, smoking, and daily calcium intake).

Two particular forms of phytoestrogen are useful in controlling menopausal symptoms. They are: isoflavones, found in soy products and red clover; and lignans found in flaxseeds. Other sources of isoflavones and lignans are shown in the box on the left. The average daily consumption of isoflavones by the Japanese from their traditional food is 50–100mg, whereas the current daily consumption in the West is less than 3mg. Interestingly, a diet high in isoflavones may benefit men, too. Scientists believe that Asian men have a reduced death rate from both prostate cancer and heart disease as a result of their isoflavone-rich diet.

ADDING PHYTOESTROGEN TO YOUR DAILY DIET

To alleviate menopausal symptoms, you should aim to eat 100mg of isoflavones each day. The best way to get enough is to consume phytoestrogen-rich foods little and often throughout the day, as isoflavones appear to leave the body quite quickly.

Foods rich in phytoestrogens, such as soy yogurts and milk, are widely available. The recipe section (see Part 2) includes many delicious dishes designed to make soy enjoyable. Here are a few examples of how you can include phytoestrogens in your daily diet.

• A sandwich made with two slices of soy and flaxseed bread. Phytoestrogen content: 22mg
• 125g/4½oz/½ cup portion of whipped soy dessert. Phytoestrogen content: 20mg
• 125g/4½oz/½ cup portion of soy yogurt. Phytoestrogen content: 10mg
• A 250ml/9fl oz glass of soy fruit shake. Phytoestrogen content: 20mg
• A 250ml/9fl oz glass of soy milk. Phytoestrogen content: 20mg
• Any recipe in Part 2 that includes 100g/3½oz tofu. Phytoestrogen content: 25mg
• A slice of soy and flaxseed fruit loaf. Phytoestrogen content: 10mg
• A Phyto-Fix Bar (see page 138). Phytoestrogen content: 10mg
• Two soy crêpes (see pages 68–9). Phytoestrogen content: 10mg
• A bowl of Phyto Muesli (see page 71) with soy milk and ground flaxseeds. Phytoestrogen content: 30mg

Keep in mind that flaxseeds are available both in ground form and seed form; if you buy the ground form, it's easy to add them to cereals, yogurts, soups, smoothies and shakes. It's thought that there are about 300 times more lignans in flaxseeds compared to sunflower seeds.

As well as including plenty of phytoestrogens in your diet, it's important to take measures to maximize their absorption. Alcohol and cigarettes both tend to impede the absorption of estrogen and it's been well documented that a course of antibiotics can also disturb absorption for several months. Reducing your alcohol consumption to only small quantities, minimizing or quitting smoking, and taking a supplement of probiotics after a course of antibiotics will help improve phytoestrogen absorption.

In addition to eating 100mg of phytoestrogens daily, your goal should be to eat an all-round healthy diet and to put back some of the nutrients that time and nature have removed, including magnesium, zinc, B vitamins and essential fatty acids. For the essential dos and don'ts of the menopause diet see pages 30–31.

FAT, FIBRE AND YOUR HORMONES

Today's diet is very different from that of our Stone Age ancestors. Three million years ago, vegetable matter, including hard seeds and plant fibre such as roots and stems, was the mainstay of their diet, rather than the large amounts of meat protein we consume today. The meat we buy from the butcher or supermarket is also much higher in fat, especially saturated fat, than the wild meat eaten by our ancestors. Research shows that the amount of fat and fibre you eat has a significant impact on your hormones. If your diet is high in animal fat and low in fibre (which is typical in the West), you're more likely to have high levels of estrogen circulating in your body. If you eat a low-fat, high fibre diet, your circulating estrogen levels are likely to be lower (dietary fibre speeds up the rate at which estrogen leaves the body).

So it may be that Western women who have followed high-fat, low-fibre diets are much more likely to experience menopausal symptoms due to estrogen withdrawal. Their bodies are used to a relatively high level of circulating estrogen. As a result, they don't tolerate the natural drop in estrogen when they reach the menopause as well as women who have low levels of circulating estrogen consistently throughout their life.

In theory, this means that making a dramatic change from your current diet to a low-fat, high-fibre diet could aggravate symptoms of estrogen withdrawal, although the effect is likely to be offset by the fact that your diet is healthier, which in turn has a positive effect on your hormone function. If you do change your diet, do so gradually. For example, don't suddenly go from being a meat-eater to following a weight-loss vegan diet.

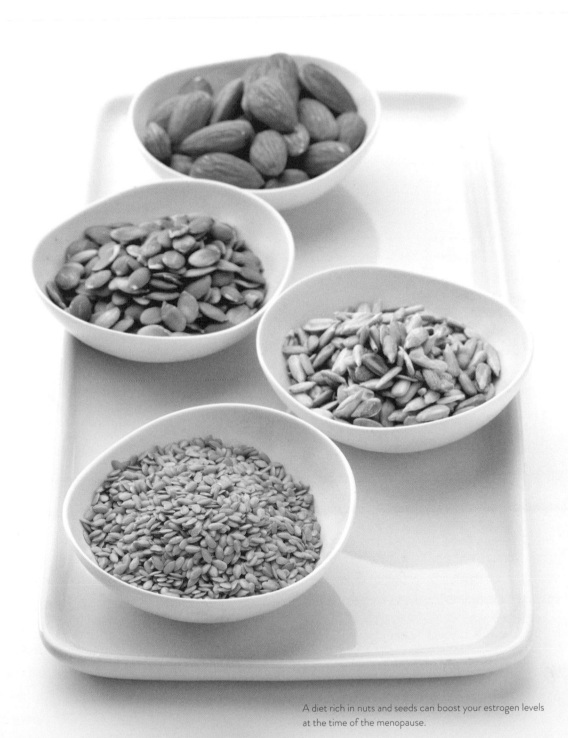

A diet rich in nuts and seeds can boost your estrogen levels at the time of the menopause.

DOS AND DON'TS OF THE NATURAL MENOPAUSE PLAN DIET

DO

◆ Eat 100mg of phytoestrogens each day. Consume foods that are rich in phytoestrogens little and often over the course of the day.

◆ Add two tablespoons of golden flaxseeds to breakfast cereal, yogurt or fruit salad. As well as being rich in phytoestrogens, they are a good source of fibre and can help constipation. They also help prevent some estrogen-dependent cancers, including prostate and ovarian cancer, and they reduce the incidence of heart problems and the bone-thinning disease osteoporosis.

◆ Eat at least five servings of fresh fruit and vegetables per day. These provide plenty of potassium and magnesium, plus small amounts of phytoestrogens. Where possible, eat organic products or grow your own.

◆ Eat foods rich in calcium and magnesium, such as milk, green leafy vegetables, unsalted nuts and seeds, wholegrains and bony fish, including sardines and whitebait.

◆ Have a serving of dairy products each day. These provide calcium and additional amounts of protein. Choose low-fat options if you need to lose weight, but avoid skimmed milk, which contains no vitamin A (semi-skimmed is preferable).

◆ Try to drink the equivalent of at least eight glasses of water daily, including herbal and fruit tea. Rooibos tea can be made with milk and is a good alternative to ordinary tea. Let hot drinks cool down, as the heat may trigger a flush.

◆ Eat regularly. Three meals a day help to ensure a good balanced diet and a steady flow of energy throughout the day.

◆ Include protein from animal or vegetarian sources in at least one meal a day. Low-protein diets jeopardize the balance of many nutrients, including calcium, vitamin B and iron.

◆ Eat three portions of oily fish per week, including salmon, mackerel, herring or sardines, which are a rich source of omega-3 fatty acids and help with hormone and joint health.

◆ Eat nutritious snacks between meals if you get hungry. Nuts, Phyto-Fix Bars (see page 138), unsalted nuts and seeds, fresh fruit or dried fruit that hasn't been dipped in sulphur dioxide are ideal.

◆ Limit your consumption of red meat to one or two portions a week. Eat fish, poultry, peas, beans and nuts instead.

DON'T

◆ Exceed national guidelines on alcohol consumption (in the UK, no more than 14 units per week; in the US, no more than one alcoholic drink per day). Ideally, limit yourself to three alcoholic drinks per week. Alcohol aggravates flushes, insomnia and, in excess, can worsen or cause many nutritional deficiencies at a time when you need to be conserving essential nutrients.

◆ Drink endless cups of coffee and tea. Caffeine can aggravate flushes, as well as anxiety and insomnia, so choose herbal alternatives instead.

◆ Eat very heavily spiced food. Hot spices, like hot drinks and alcohol, can bring on flushes.

◆ Eat sugar and junk food, including sugar added to tea and coffee, sweets, cakes, biscuits, chocolate, jam, marmalade, honey, ice cream and soft drinks containing phosphates. They may reduce the uptake of essential nutrients, and cause water retention and bloating.

◆ Add salt to your cooking or at the table, as we already have far more salt than we need from hidden sources. Avoid salted foods like kippers and bacon. Salt causes fluid retention and encourages calcium loss from the body in your urine. Use potassium-rich salt substitutes or other flavourings such as garlic, onion, kelp powder, fresh herbs, sesame powder or other mild spices.

◆ Go shopping on an empty stomach otherwise you may be tempted to fill your basket with the high-fat, calorie-laden foods you're supposed to be avoiding.

◆ Eat foods containing wheat and bran in the short term if you feel bloated or experience wind or constipation.

◆ Eat lots of fatty food. Limit your intake of fats to no more than 30 percent of your dietary intake. For most of us, this means reducing our consumption by at least 25 percent. Avoid hydrogenated fats and anything other than small amounts of butter. Instead choose cold-pressed oils, including sunflower, sesame and safflower, as well as olive oil.

◆ Smoke cigarettes – they aggravate hot flushes and night sweats, and can bring on an earlier menopause. If you do smoke, try to pace yourself between cigarettes and cut down gradually until you can manage to quit altogether.

THE NATURAL MENOPAUSE PLAN SUPPLEMENTS

However healthily you eat, sometimes it just isn't possible to achieve the desired balance of nutrients through diet alone. That's why I recommend supplements to improve your overall health. Specific supplements can also be very effective at reducing menopausal symptoms such as hot flushes and night sweats. Look at the chart on pages 34 to 35 to decide which supplements are right for you.

You're probably already familiar with vitamin and mineral, and fish oil supplements, but you may be less aware of some of the other supplements I use in the Natural Menopause Plan. In particular Femenessence (a maca root supplement), which you can read about in detail on page 37, and isoflavone-rich supplements (see below). As I described on page 26, isoflavones act as an alternative to HRT by giving you a boost of plant estrogens. If your menopausal symptoms are severe, a combination of a phytoestrogen-rich diet and isoflavone-rich supplements can bring the best results in the shortest time. Before we used estrogen-moderating supplements in our Natural Menopause Plan, it used to take at least three or four months to control hot flushes. Once we included supplements, women began returning for their follow-up appointment (within one month), delighted that both their hot flushes and night sweats were far milder.

Women often ask whether they need to take isoflavone-rich supplements indefinitely. The answer depends on the amount of isoflavones you have in your diet. If you enjoy eating soy and settle into a routine, you may require fewer isoflavone-rich supplements. However, research suggests it's advisable to continue with an isoflavone-rich regime for life to protect your bones, heart and cognitive function. The two main isoflavone-rich supplements you can buy are described below.

RED CLOVER SUPPLEMENTS

Red clover is the richest known source of four important estrogenic isoflavones. It has up to ten times as much of these isoflavones as the next richest source, soy. In studies, red clover has been shown to dramatically improve night sweats, hot flushes and vaginal atrophy. And it's not associated with some of the complications of HRT, such as thickening of the womb lining, adverse effects on breast tissue and weight gain. I recommend Promensil as a first-line treatment – this is a standardized red clover supplement made by Novogen. Each 500mg tablet of Promensil is designed to deliver the same dose of isoflavones as a vegetarian diet based on pulses/legumes (approximately 40mg of the four isoflavones). Taking red clover in pill form is the only way you're likely to get an adequate amount, especially if you don't digest soy well.

PHYTO SOY SUPPLEMENTS

This is another phytoestrogen supplement I recommend. A clinical trial showed that phyto soy capsules can reduce hot flushes and other bothersome menopausal symptoms such as insomnia, anxiety, mood problems and loss of libido. There are many soy isoflavone supplements on the market, but they vary in quality. I recommend Phyto Soya capsules by Arkopharma. They are standardized and come in two strengths (17.5mg and 35mg of isoflavones per capsule). You probably won't need to take *both* Promensil (red clover) and phyto soy supplements. Try taking Promensil first (in conjunction with a soy-rich diet), and add phyto soy only if your flushes and other symptoms persist. You can also take both supplements if you don't tolerate soy in your diet well, or if you're away from home and can't follow your usual soy-based diet.

GUIDELINES FOR TAKING ALL SUPPLEMENTS

- *Choose standardized supplements. "Standardized" supplements are prepared to pharmaceutical standards and have undergone clinical trials.*
- *Buy supplements from a reputable source. Most of the supplements I recommend are available in health-food shops (see page 158 for a list of stockists).*
- *Start by taking supplements gradually. For example, if it's recommended you take two to four capsules of a supplement a day, start by taking one tablet per day and gradually build up to the optimum dose over a week or two.*
- *Supplements should always be taken after meals, unless otherwise specified.*
- *Most of the supplements suggested on pages 34–35 are compatible with medication; however, you should consult your doctor before taking St John's wort if you are taking prescribed medication. Also, if you're taking prescribed drugs, don't reduce the dose without your doctor's agreement.*
- *How long you continue to take your supplements is up to you. Supplements that are being taken to address certain symptoms can be reduced gradually once your symptoms are under control. If you reduce your supplement dose too quickly and symptoms return, increase the dosage again.*
- *If you're taking supplements to prevent osteoporosis, bear in mind that you're most at risk of bone loss during the first five years after the menopause. Although bone loss slows down in the following ten years, it's still significant. So if you are at risk of osteoporosis, you may need to take supplements for some time, while also having a bone density scan every few years to check your bone mass.*

CHOOSING YOUR SUPPLEMENTS

PROBLEM	SUPPLEMENT, COMMENTS AND DOSAGE
General symptoms of the menopause	Take Femenessence (maca root) to improve your hormonal balance and alleviate general menopausal symptoms. Take 2 x 500mg capsules twice daily (morning and evening). Also take a good-quality vitamin and mineral supplement designed for your age group. I recommend Fema 45+ (2 capsules a day), Gynocite (2 capsules a day) or Blackmores Proactive Multi 50+ (2–3 capsules a day).
Hot flushes and night sweats	Take Promensil (a red clover supplement). Take 1 tablet a day, which delivers 40mg of isoflavones. Also follow a phytoestrogen-rich diet. If Promensil doesn't bring you symptom relief (or if you can't eat a phytoestrogen-rich diet for any reason), add in Arkopharma Phyto Soya capsules. You can also take Arkopharma Phyto Soya by itself if Promensil doesn't suit you. Take 1–2 capsules a day, providing 17.5mg isoflavones per capsule. You can also take higher-strength capsules (35mg isoflavones per capsule), but see if your symptoms respond to the lower strength first. Femenessence (see above) has also been shown to help. You can also take sage leaf for hot flushes, but try phytoestrogen supplements first. Take 300–900mg sage tablets a day.
Vaginal dryness	Take omega-7 (sea buckthorn oil); 2 capsules twice a day. This will alleviate bleeding during sex and vaginal dryness. Also use Arkopharma Phyto Soya Vaginal Gel; insert this twice a week at bedtime.
Lack of sex drive	Take a supplement called ArginMax (a combination of herbs, vitamins, minerals and the amino acid L-arginine), which enhances circulation and sexual arousal. Take three in the morning and three at night. If you can't access ArginMax, try taking horny goat weed tablets instead; 600mg a day.

PROBLEM	SUPPLEMENT, COMMENTS AND DOSAGE
Lack of sex drive combined with depression	Take St John's wort; 900mg a day. *Caution*: if you are taking prescribed medication, consult your doctor before taking St John's wort.
Heavy periods	Take a magnesium citrate supplement; 2 x 150mg tablets daily. Also take iron – ferrous sulphate; 1 x 200mg tablet daily with fruit juice. Vitex agnus castus can also help with heavy periods; take 1,000mg a day.
Painful periods	Take a magnesium supplement; 150–300mg daily (magnesium supplements can cause loose stools, so lower your daily dose if you have this side-effect). Also take an evening primrose oil supplement; 2,000–4,000iu a day.
Depression	Take St John's wort; 900mg a day. See caution above.
Insomnia	Take valerian tablets; 600mg at bedtime.
General aches and pains (especially joint pain)	Take glucosamine sulphate and chondroitin; 400mg three times a day. High-strength fish oil; 750mg twice a day. Or take Regenovex capsules; 1 a day.
Dry skin	Apply Arkopharma Phyto Soya Face Cream and body lotion daily.
Osteoporosis	Take a vitamin and mineral complex containing calcium, magnesium and vitamin D (follow dosage directions on the packaging). Also take Promensil (red clover); 1 tablet a day. Or Femenessence Macapause; 2 x 500mg capsules twice daily.

THE NATURAL MENOPAUSE PLAN THERAPIES

Several complementary therapies work very well in treating menopausal symptoms such as hot flushes and night sweats. They can also make you feel better overall, acting as an antidote to the stresses and strains of life, and making you feel like you're back in the driver's seat.

Whichever complementary therapy you choose, it's important to put yourself in the hands of an experienced and qualified practitioner. Recognized complementary therapies have official associations that keep registers of qualified practitioners. You can contact these practitioners locally or ask for a recommendation in your local health food store.

HERBAL MEDICINE

Herbal medicine has been used for thousands of years to help treat common conditions. In our NHAS survey of midlife women, 24 percent of women had tried herbs and, of these, 80 percent

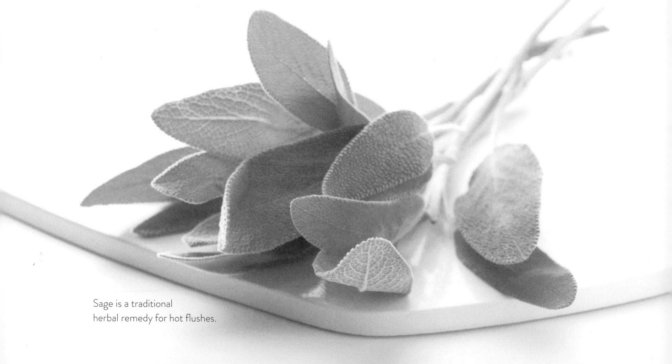

Sage is a traditional
herbal remedy for hot flushes.

had found them useful. Many herbs have now undergone clinical trials to examine how they work and why. The following herbs are those that are most commonly used and successful in treating menopausal symptoms.

Peruvian maca root This is the main herbal remedy I use in the Natural Menopause Plan for general menopausal symptoms. In particular I recommend a supplement called Femenessence, which I consider to be a safe natural alternative to HRT. Femenessence is the first herbal product made from maca root (maca is a plant native to the highlands of Peru) that has been shown in trials to raise estrogen and progesterone levels – the two key hormones that fall at the time of the perimenopause. Clinical trials show it can bring about an 84 percent reduction in menopausal symptoms. Women report fewer hot flushes and night sweats, and improved sleep, energy levels, mood and libido. Femenessence works by stimulating the hormone-secreting glands in the body, such as the pituitary and adrenal glands. In the process it also has a positive impact on your cholesterol levels (see page 47) and bone health. There are two types of Femenessence: one for perimenopausal women (MacaLife)and one for postmenopausal women (MacaPause). Dosage: 2 x 500mg capsules twice daily (morning and evening).

Licorice root Also known as *Glycyrrhiza glabra* and sarsaparilla root, this contains phytoestrogens. It can be used in conjunction with other herbs and brewed into a herbal tea. However, licorice can cause sodium retention and increases the risk of high blood pressure in some people. If you are one of a very small minority of women whose symptoms don't respond to the Natural Menopause Plan after six months, consult a herbalist about taking this herb.

Dong quai Also known as *Angelica polymorphia*, this contains phytoestrogens and is considered in Chinese medicine to be a harmonizing tonic. It has traditionally been used to treat female complaints, such as heavy bleeding and premenstrual syndrome (PMS). As with licorice root, consult a herbalist about taking dong quai if other phytoestrogen supplements haven't worked for you

Sage leaf Also known as *Salvia officianalis*, this member of the mint family contains estrogenic substances that help to relieve hot flushes and night sweats. Try taking sage if you've already tried Promensil (a red clover supplement) and phyto soy capsules and they haven't helped your hot flushes. Dosage: 300–900mg in tablet form once a day.

Vitex agnus castus   Research has found this can significantly relieve PMS symptoms, such as irritability, mood swings, headaches, breast fullness, abdominal cramps and depression. It can also help with heavy periods. Results are usually noticeable within three cycles. Dosage: 1,000mg in tablet form once a day.

Horny goat weed   Also known as *Epimedium*, this plant has aphrodisiac properties and can help to revive a dwindling sex drive. Dosage: 600mg in tablet once a day.

Valerian   This is a traditional herbal remedy for the relief of stress and tension, and it promotes natural sleep without the unpleasant side-effects of conventional sleeping pills. It can also be taken for anxiety and conditions that are worsened by stress, such as irritable bowel syndrome. Dosage: 600mg in tablet form at night.

Panax ginseng   This is moderately helpful in controlling hot flushes, especially in conjunction with natural vitamin E. Consult a herbalist about taking it if other phytoestrogen supplements haven't worked for you. ·

St John's wort   Also known as Hypericum, this herb has been used to treat depression for many years. It's thought to be most effective in treating moderate depression and has fewer side-effects than conventional antidepressants. It may also help increase libido. If you're taking prescribed drugs, check with your doctor before taking St John's wort. Dosage: 900mg in tablet form once a day.

Black cohosh   Black cohosh has been a promising herbal supplement for the reduction of menopausal symptoms such as hot flushes and night sweats. However, it's unsuitable for women with a family history of breast cancer and, in the past, there has been debate about its impact on liver health. For these reasons, I tend not to recommend black cohosh as a first-line treatment. However, if the other treatments I recommend for menopausal symptoms haven't worked for you, consult a herbalist about the possibility of taking black cohosh.

HOMEOPATHY

The word homeopathy comes from the Greek *homoeo* (meaning "similar") and *pathos* (meaning "suffering"). It's designed to produce the same symptoms from which you are suffering. This is said to stimulate the body to fight back against them. The dosages are very small and often only contain an energy or "spirit" of the original medicine. Several small studies have suggested that homeopathy may help women with menopausal symptoms, including hot flushes, fatigue and mood disturbances. However, more research is required to accurately determine the benefits of homeopathy.

Sepia and sulphur are two of the many remedies that may be indicated for hot flushes and night sweats. Try taking either of these remedies – they should be available in health food stores (follow the dosage directions on the packaging).

There is also a wide choice of homeopathic remedies for poor memory, depression, insomnia, anxiety attacks, irritability, headaches and confusion. Seek advice from a homeopath about remedies that are tailored to your individual needs.

ACUPUNCTURE AND ACUPRESSURE

Many problems that occur at the time of the menopause may respond to acupuncture. This treatment uses fine needles inserted at specific points in your body, known as meridians, to help to unblock energy channels. It's not uncommon for energy in the body to become blocked, leading to all manner of symptoms from irritability and anxiety to insomnia and headaches. Acupressure, which involves applying pressure at certain points on your body with your fingertips, can also be a useful self-help tool.

TRY LETTING GO...

If you're suffering from frequent hot flushes or feelings of stress and anxiety, try this simple letting-go exercise once a day. It releases muscle tension and can quickly make you feel better.

1 Wear loose clothes and find a warm, quiet place where you won't be interrupted. Put on some calming music to help you to relax, and adjust the lighting so it's not too bright. Lie down with a pillow beneath your head. Instead of focusing on the outside world, tune in to your body and become aware of any tension.

2 Relax your arms, shoulders and lower jaw. Take a few slow, deep breaths.

3 Concentrate on tensing and then fully relaxing your muscles, starting with your feet, then gradually working your way up your legs, torso and arms. Finish with your neck, head and face. When your whole body feels relaxed, lie quietly for 15 minutes.

4 Gradually allow yourself to come to. Roll onto your side, sit up slowly and sip a glass of water.

CRANIAL OSTEOPATHY

Cranial osteopathy involves gentle manipulation of the body's soft tissues. It can help with long-standing back, head and neck problems and has been shown to reduce hot flushes. Treatment for women suffering menopausal symptoms is often aimed at improving function of the pituitary gland. This gland, found at the base of the brain, balances the function of the adrenal glands and consequently many of the body's functions.

RELAXATION THERAPIES

Stress can have a negative effect on your overall health and wellbeing, and more specifically can exacerbate symptoms such as hot flushes and night sweats. If you dedicate time every day to relaxing and recharging your batteries, the effects can be extremely beneficial. Research shows that 15–20 minutes of relaxation a day can reduce hot flushes by up to 60 percent. Given the fast pace of our lives and the difficulty of taking time out, relaxation is often hard to achieve. This is why it helps to explore formal relaxation therapies. The following four therapies are particularly soothing.

PICTURE YOURSELF SOMEWHERE BEAUTIFUL

This creative visualization exercise is an enjoyable way to relax, and is ideal if you don't have enough time for yoga or Pilates. Creative visualization does require practice and you may have to work at it before you feel the full benefits. If your mind is very busy, try to clear it by writing down your thoughts first.

1 Wear loose clothes and find a warm, quiet place where you won't be interrupted. Lie down on the floor with a pillow under your head.
2 Bend your knees, keeping your feet flat on the floor. Close your eyes, breathing steadily and slowly. Consciously relax your face, fingers, arms, legs and toes.
3 Start to visualize yourself in a beautiful place – anything from a boat on a sparkling blue sea to a peaceful garden full of flowers. Keep your mind focused on your fantasy for as long as you can. Bring it to life by imagining the smells, sounds and sights you would witness. Make it as rich in detail as possible. After 15–20 minutes, bring yourself gently back to reality, rolling onto your side before you stand up.

Creative visualization As well as being a tool for relaxation, creative visualization can help you to think more positively about yourself. By creating a mental picture of yourself in a pleasurable environment, or by picturing yourself as contented, self-confident and optimistic, you can achieve more happiness and positivity in your life. Try taking 5–10 minutes out each day to visualize yourself the way you would like to be. Experts believe that the best time for this is first thing in the morning and last thing at night, so start and finish your day by imagining yourself in great physical and mental shape with good things happening to you. Picture yourself having fun with your partner or with a friend, or perhaps starting a new relationship. Or perhaps your daydreams will centre on success in your work or even fulfilling a lifetime ambition.

Whatever you decide to focus on, make the images in your mind so realistic that you actually start to feel you are experiencing the situation. It may take some practice, but once you get the hang of it, it will become like watching a movie. Remember that unless you **feel** positive about yourself, you don't stand much chance of people reacting in a positive way toward you. Visualization is an acquired skill, so if your mind keeps wandering, stick with it – eventually you will get it. You have nothing to lose and it's a positive way to begin and end each day. Start now with the exercise in the box on the left.

Guided relaxation When you're feeling anxious and tired, it can help to use a power napping tool (see page 158) or to listen to a guided relaxation. The latter will take you step by step through specific techniques that will turn your attention inward and help you to achieve full-body relaxation. Try the guided meditation on my *Get Fit for Midlife* DVD (see page 158) at bedtime

Yoga Yoga has been practised for thousands of years. It works on the principle that mind, body and soul need to be working in perfect harmony for optimal health. To help you achieve this, yoga uses asanas (postures that relax muscles) and pranayama (breathing techniques that help improve the oxygen flow in your body and regulate your breathing). Yogic meditation and relaxation exercises help to still the mind. Attend a yoga class to learn the basic postures, then practise at home on a regular basis.

Pilates Pilates is a more recent relaxation therapy that also exercises the body. Developed in the 1920s, this combination of Eastern and Western philosophies teaches you breathing techniques with movement, body mechanics, balance, coordination, positioning of the body, spatial awareness, strength and flexibility. As with yoga, you should first go to some classes to learn the exercises before practising them at home.

BUILD YOUR BONES

After the menopause, women become more vulnerable to osteoporosis, a condition in which the bones become brittle and less able to absorb shock. Eventually the bones can weaken so much that even a small knock or fall can cause a fracture.

So what causes osteoporosis? You may not think of your bones as living tissue, but they go through a constant process of renewal during our lives. Until the age of 35, we make as much new bone as we lose, keeping the scales in balance. But from then on, we tend to lose around 1 percent of our total bone mass each year until we reach the menopause. From that point, bone loss accelerates at a further 2–3 percent per year for up to ten years.

This is partly due to falling levels of estrogen, as one of the key roles of this important hormone is to maintain bone mass. But genetics and lifestyle are also involved. Experts think that the level of bone density we lay down in our lifetime is 70 percent due to genetic factors and 30 percent due to lifestyle factors, such as diet, exercise and how much we drink and smoke. By learning to meet your needs at midlife, you can stimulate the growth of new bone naturally.

ASSESS YOUR RISK

Answer "yes" or "no" to these questions:

- In your childhood and teens, did you consume a poor diet, low in calcium (especially dairy products)?
- Do you regularly consume red meat, rather than including vegetarian sources of protein in your diet?
- Did you experience an early menopause, spontaneously or following surgery?
- Do you have a history of thyroid or other hormonal problems?
- Have you been underweight or suffered an eating disorder, such as anorexia or bulimia?
- Have you always had a petite build?
- Do you smoke ten or more cigarettes per day?
- Have there been times in your life when you regularly drank alcohol in excess of national guidelines (see page 31)?
- Do you only rarely perform formal weight-bearing exercise?
- Do you lead a sedentary lifestyle?
- Have you had periods of excessive physical activity in your life, for example, as an athlete or dancer?
- Have you taken steroid drugs for an extended period of time?

• *Have you suffered more than one fracture since your menopause?*

• *Has a close relative suffered from osteoporosis?*

• *Have you experienced a chronic illness that affected your digestion, kidney and liver function?*

• *Did you ever stop having periods, especially when you were young?*

If you answered "yes" to just one of these questions, you have a higher than average risk of osteoporosis. If you answered "yes" to more than two questions, start the preventive measures below as soon as possible.

EAT FOODS THAT PRESERVE BONE HEALTH

A diet rich in calcium helps to preserve your bone mass, but it's not the only factor. Magnesium, phosphorous, boron and vitamins C and D are also important. In particular, magnesium helps the body to absorb and use calcium. Getting a healthy balance of these two minerals is vital.

Include dairy products in your diet on a daily basis – they are dense sources of calcium. But also eat plenty of green, leafy vegetables such as watercress, kale, broccoli or cabbage, because this provides the perfect balance of calcium and magnesium. Nuts and seeds also provide balanced amounts of these two minerals.

Eating dairy products and green, leafy vegetables in your everyday diet provides the right balance of calcium and magnesium for your bones.

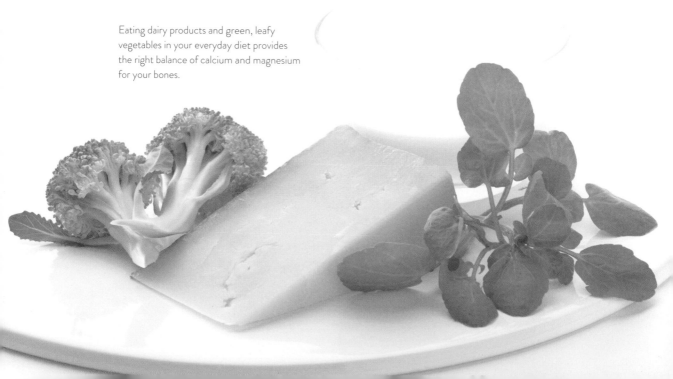

Vitamin D also helps your body to absorb calcium. The action of sunlight on your skin provides the main source. During the summer expose your face and arms to the sun without sunscreen (but take care not to burn) for 8–12 minutes a day if you have fair to medium skin, or 45 minutes a day if you have dark skin. If you spend longer in the sun, apply sunscreen with a sun protection factor (SPF) of at least 15. Small amounts of vitamin D can be found in some foods, mainly egg yolk and oily fish.

Research suggests that foods rich in omega-3 and omega-6 essential fatty acids help the absorption of calcium from food. Omega-3s are found in fish oil supplements, oily fish (salmon, mackerel, herring, sardines and pilchards) and some cooking oils, such as rapeseed and flaxseed. Good sources of omega-6s include sunflower and corn oils, almonds, green leafy vegetables, flaxseeds and wholegrain cereals.

Make sure your diet includes plenty of plant phytoestrogen (see page 26). Good sources include soy beans, soy products such as tofu and soy milk, flaxseeds and, to a lesser degree, lentils, chickpeas and mung beans. Femenessence (maca root; see page 37) has also been shown to regenerate new bone.

LIMIT OR AVOID CERTAIN FOODS

There are also some foods you should limit in your diet. Try not to have too much meat protein, salt or caffeine, as excessive quantities can reduce your body's ability to absorb and retain calcium. Excessive alcohol is also thought to interfere with calcium metabolism and affect bone-building cells, resulting in loss of bone density.

DO WEIGHT-BEARING EXERCISE

Exercise plays a vital part in keeping bones healthy. High-impact activities are the most beneficial. Running, jogging, brisk walking and lifting weights are all good choices. You can lift weights in a gym with weight-training equipment or at home using free weights.

As you age, gentler alternatives include golf, gardening and dancing. Pilates and yoga are also good weight-bearing exercises. We repeatedly see good production of new bone in patients not taking HRT, but it does take several years to notice the difference on a bone density scan. Nine years ago, my own bone mass measured average for my age, which was quite a shock as I expected it to be higher. Five years later, after doing regular weight-bearing exercise for over four years, I had another bone density scan and was delighted to find that my bone mass was now 17 percent above average.

Aim for at least 30–45 minutes of moderate exercise at least 4–5 times a week. Build up gradually. Start with the strengthening exercises in the box opposite. Do these daily or at least five times a week; they target the key body parts that are vulnerable to fractures.

EXERCISES TO BUILD BONE MASS

Upper spine

1 Lie flat on your back on the floor or on a bed. Press your head backward and push for a count of five. Release and repeat. Don't hold your breath (counting out loud can help), since this can increase your blood pressure.

2 Now lie on your front, preferably on a hard surface. Squeeze your shoulder blades together, then try to lift your head and shoulders straight up a short way off the floor. Lower and repeat a few times. Gradually increase the number of repetitions. Don't bend your neck backward – keep looking at the floor at all times so your spine remains in a straight line.

3 Move to a seated position, pull your shoulder blades together and hold briefly. Repeat 10 times.

Hips

1 Standing on one leg, lift your other leg out to the side in a smooth, controlled manner, then lower it back down. Repeat 10–15 times, then swap legs.

2 Make sure you stand upright throughout the movement and don't allow the supporting hip to push out to the side to compensate. This exercise can also be performed while lying on your side with your upper leg moving in a vertical plane.

3 Alternatively, lie on your back with your knees bent and your legs positioned on the inside of the legs of a chair. Try to push your knees and legs apart (the chair legs will prevent this). Hold for a count of five, then release. Remember not to hold your breath.

Ankles

1 Stand upright, gently leaning against a chair or bench, and lift your heels off the floor.

2 Check that your ankles do not roll outward and keep your weight over your big toes.

Wrists

1 Stand an arm's length from a wall, arms straight out, with your hands flat on the wall at shoulder height.

2 Slowly bend your elbows, bringing your face and chest closer to the wall, then pushing back out (like doing a push-up against the wall). Repeat 10–15 times.

3 As you become more proficient, you can perform this exercise on the floor on your hands and knees: gradually lower your body toward the floor, keeping your back straight.

GET HEART HEALTHY

You may think of heart disease as predominantly a male problem. Indeed, before the menopause, your risk is much lower than for men of the same age (estrogen protects you). However, after the menopause, your risk of atherosclerosis (furring and hardening of the arteries), high blood pressure, angina, heart attack and stroke becomes similar to that of men. Thirty percent of postmenopausal women will develop heart disease.

It seems that the menopause brings changes in the level of blood fats known as lipids, which determine your cholesterol level. There are two components of cholesterol: high-density lipoproteins (HDLs), which have a beneficial, cleansing effect in the bloodstream, and low-density lipoproteins (LDLs), which encourage fat and mineral deposits, known as plaque, to accumulate on the walls of arteries, causing them to narrow and clog up.

In postmenopausal women, as a direct result of estrogen deficiency, LDL cholesterol appears to increase, while HDL decreases. An elevated LDL and total cholesterol level is linked to a higher risk of stroke, heart attack and death.

The good news is that heart disease isn't inevitable – there are lots of preventative measures you can take. According to research in 1990 at the University of California, diet can be as effective in combating atherosclerosis as drugs or surgery. A group of people with severely blocked arteries went on a very low-fat vegetarian diet and an exercise and meditation programme – at the end their arteries were found to be clear of plaque.

ASSESS YOUR RISK

Answer "yes" or "no" to these questions:

• *Do you smoke?*

• *Do you exercise less than 3–4 times a week?*

• *Do you eat a lot of fatty foods, such as hamburgers and red meat?*

• *Are you overweight?*

• *Do you have high blood pressure?*

• *Is your cholesterol count high?*

• *Do you drink more than the recommended safe limits of alcohol (see page 31)?*

• *Do you eat fish, especially oily fish, less than twice a week?*

• *Do you eat less than five portions of fruit and vegetables a day?*

If you answered "yes" to more than three questions, try making the following changes.

FOLLOW A HEART-HEALTHY DIET

It's been known for years that the saturated fats found mainly in animal protein, such as meat, dairy products and eggs, can contribute to atherosclerosis, so you should cut down on fatty foods such as burgers, sausages and pies.

But this doesn't mean that you need to cut out fat completely. Monounsaturated fats, found in olive oil and rapeseed/canola oil, and polyunsaturated fatty acids, derived from a variety of plants, flaxseeds, fish oils and cold-pressed flaxseed oil, can shift the balance toward the good HDL cholesterol (although the degree of protection these "healthy" oils offer is still debated). Include oily fish, such as salmon, mackerel, herring, sardines and pilchards, in your diet at least twice a week. Omega-3 fatty acids in these fish can help to protect against heart and circulatory disease. As part of a heart-healthy lifestyle, you should also eat at least five portions of fruit and vegetables every day. Add chopped fruit to breakfast cereals and snack on fruit and vegetables throughout the day. As well as helping to prevent heart disease, this will help you to control your weight – fruit and vegetables are filling but relatively low in calories.

Several studies over the past few decades show that including soy in your diet may help to protect against heart disease by lowering cholesterol levels. It was discovered almost by accident in the late 1960s that soy protein has a cholesterol-lowering effect. Researchers who were looking at whether soy could be a palatable alternative protein to meat discovered a marked reduction in cholesterol levels in people who consumed a lot of soy products.

In 1999, the US Food and Drug Administration (FDA) approved a health claim for soy protein and its role in reducing the risk of coronary heart disease. This same endorsement was eventually granted by the UK authorities. This means that it can be stated on the label of food products containing at least 6.25mg of soy protein per serving that the product may reduce the risk of heart disease when consumed in conjunction with a low-fat, low-cholesterol diet. To increase your intake of soya products, try drinking soy milk on a daily basis and try out the delicious recipes containing soy in Part 2 (see page 62).

In addition to eating a heart-healthy diet, you may like to take a supplement called Femenessence, which is made from Peruvian maca root (see page 37). As well as stimulating the hormone-secreting glands in the body (and easing menopausal symptoms), Femenessence also lowers the level of bad LDL cholesterol and raises the level of good HDL cholesterol in your body.

AVOID FOODS THAT CAN DAMAGE YOUR HEART

Apart from cutting down on saturated fat, it's important to make sure you don't consume more than a teaspoon or 6g of salt a day. There's a well-documented link between eating too much salt and high blood pressure, which in turn increases your risk of developing coronary heart disease. To cut down on salt, avoid adding it to food either during cooking or at the table. Also be aware of hidden salt in foods such as packaged soups and sauces, baked beans and canned vegetables, pizzas and other convenience foods. Even some breakfast cereals contain salt. Get into the habit of checking food labels for salt content before you buy a product.

Limit the amount of alcohol you drink too: drinking more than the recommended limits (see page 31) can also cause high blood pressure. And because alcohol is high in calories it can lead to weight gain – obesity is another risk factor for heart disease.

DO REGULAR AEROBIC EXERCISE

Regular aerobic exercise, such as walking, swimming or cycling, at least five days a week will help to keep your heart and circulation in good shape. Aim for 30 minutes a day, but divide this up into 15-minute bursts if you prefer.

Exert yourself enough to feel warm and slightly breathless, but still able to hold a conversation. If you're unfit, start gently by taking regular walks and gradually increase to a level you feel comfortable with. If you're unaccustomed to exercise, just aim to increase your level of daily physical activity to start with.

- *Leave your car at home and walk to the supermarket or to work.*
- *Go for a 20-minute walk at lunchtime.*
- *Listen to your favourite music and get dancing.*
- *Take the stairs instead of the elevator.*
- *Walk up escalators.*
- *Get more active around the house and garden: vacuuming, mowing the lawn, sweeping, raking leaves and washing the car will all add to the amount of time you are physically active during the day.*
- *Enjoy active days out at the weekend: go to the beach or country and walk, swim or cycle.*

QUIT SMOKING

It is vital to stop smoking for the sake of your heart. Smoke-damaged arteries attract fatty deposits that restrict the blood flow to your heart muscle. Smoking can also make blood more sticky and likely to clot, which can lead to a blockage in an artery and a heart attack.

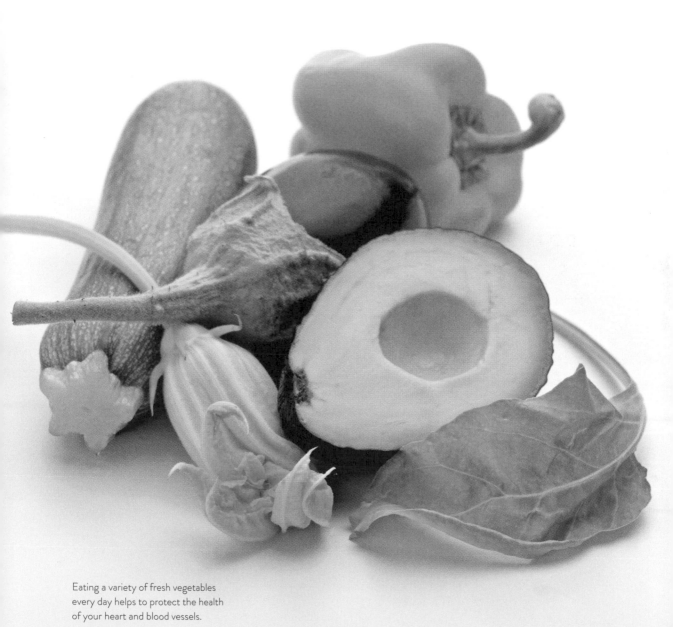

Eating a variety of fresh vegetables
every day helps to protect the health
of your heart and blood vessels.

STAY PHYSICALLY ACTIVE

Exercise becomes very important as you get older because your metabolism (the rate at which your body burns calories) tends to slow down. Exercise helps you maintain a healthy weight in several ways. Firstly, you burn calories while you're doing it, and it can also increase your metabolic rate for up to 24 hours afterwards. Secondly, regular exercise, particularly strength or resistance training, builds muscle. The greater your muscle mass, the higher your metabolic rate and the more calories you burn.

Exercise has other benefits, too. It improves the health of your heart, circulation and bones, and it lowers your blood pressure and risk of diabetes. Within 12 weeks of starting an exercise regime, you will feel more energetic, cope more effectively with stress and anxiety, sleep better, fight off infections more successfully, have better reaction times and coordination, and generally feel a whole lot better.

ASSESS YOUR FITNESS

Answer "yes" or "no" to the following questions:

• Do you exercise?

• Are you currently doing some exercise occasionally?

• Do you exercise more than three times a week for more than 30 minutes at a time?

• Does it take a lot of exercise before you feel puffed?

• Can you run up and down stairs without panting?

If you answered "no" to more than two of these questions, follow the guidelines below for becoming more active.

WHICH TYPE OF EXERCISE?

Aim to build up your activity levels slowly. If you're overweight or haven't exercised in a long time, try the gentle methods on page 48 or choose something you enjoy. If you already like walking on a treadmill or along a country lane, this is a great place to start. As you begin to feel fitter, you can take up more intense forms of exercise. Think back to activities you enjoyed when you were younger, such as tennis, swimming or dancing. Other good options include running, cycling, cardiovascular machines at the gym, squash, badminton and rope-skipping.

If you like to exercise with others, try joining an aerobics-based exercise or dance class or going for a jog with a friend. Or use your lunch hour to exercise with colleagues. If you like to exercise alone, select a good home exercise DVD or simply dance to your favourite music. It's a good idea to vary the type of exercise you do on different days of the week to target different parts of your body and prevent boredom.

HOW MUCH AND HOW OFTEN?

Start your exercise routine slowly, otherwise you risk discomfort or injury, especially if you're not used to exercise. The general consensus is that women entering the menopause and beyond should aim to exercise regularly 4–5 times a week for 30–60 minutes (provided they don't suffer from cardiovascular disease). If you prefer to exercise in short bursts of 10–15 minutes several times a day, that's fine. Build up your exercise programme gradually over at least three months. And make sure that you don't over-exercise as this can be bad for you, putting a strain on your joints and bones.

EXERCISE SAFELY

If you haven't exercised for a long time, check with your doctor before you start. This also applies if you have heart disease, high blood pressure, joint problems, back problems, are very overweight, have a serious illness or are convalescing. If it's OK to begin, make sure you follow these guidelines:

- *Before performing any exercises in your home or in your garden, check that the location is safe and that the surfaces are not wet or slippery.*
- *Make sure you are warm enough – choose layered, loose clothing that can be discarded as you heat up.*
- *Make sure the support and equipment that you use is strong enough to take your weight.*
- *Don't exercise for at least an hour after meals, and make sure you drink plenty of water to avoid becoming dehydrated.*
- *Remember to warm up. This helps to get you in the mood and also encourages blood flow to your muscles, providing oxygen to fuel your activities. You need to move your joints through their full range of movement to loosen them up and to gently stretch the muscles you are about to use. Hold stretches for 6–8 seconds, and avoid bouncing if you can. Walking, gentle jogging, marching on the spot, cycling or any activity that uses your large muscle groups are good warm-ups.*
- *Remember to cool down gradually, rather than stopping suddenly. Gently stretch the muscles that you have been using to keep them flexible. Build in some relaxation time at the end of your session to reward yourself for your efforts and to give you time to release tension.*

BEAT THE BLOAT

At the time of the menopause, our nutrient levels often become unacceptably low. As a result, our immune system, which protects us from toxins, often struggles to work efficiently. Our impaired immune system perceives certain foods and drinks as "toxic", leading to all manner of symptoms from constipation and bloating to fatigue and depression. The good news is that these conditions can usually be reversed over a few months by improving our nutrient levels.

Transient food sensitivities cause many women to produce antibodies to some foods and drinks. This process can result in water retention, as the brain instructs the cells to retain fluid in an attempt to dilute the so-called toxins. The most common temporary sensitivity is to whole wheat and grains, such as wheat, oats, barley, rye and bran. When these are excluded from your diet for a month or two, it can lead to rapid weight loss as the redundant fluid is passed.

ASSESS YOUR SYMPTOMS

Answer "yes" or "no" to the following questions.

- *Do you suffer from constipation?*
- *Do you feel bloated after eating?*
- *Do you suffer from excessive wind?*
- *Is diarrhoea a problem?*
- *Do you feel tired and depressed?*
- *Do you feel anxious for no apparent reason?*
- *Do you suffer from irritable bowel syndrome (IBS)?*

If you answered "yes" to more than two of these questions, you may have a temporary intolerance to grains, in which case you should cut them out of your diet for a while. These guidelines will help you.

ELIMINATE THE CULPRITS

Stop eating wheat, oats, barley, rye and bran for at least four weeks, and preferably for six weeks. Most supermarkets and health food stores sell a wide range of wheat-free breads, crackers, pasta, pizza bases, muffins, cakes and biscuits.

After 4–6 weeks, if your symptoms have improved, start to reintroduce the various grains one by one back into your diet. For example, choose one grain, such as rye in the form of rye crackers. As you reintroduce each grain, look out for any of these reactions: diarrhoea, constipation, excessive wind, abdominal bloating, headaches, irritability, weight gain, confusion, depression, mouth ulcers, skin rash and palpitations.

If you have no reaction after five days, choose another grain and repeat the process. Don't mix the grains because if you do experience an adverse reaction, you won't know which grain caused it. It's best to reintroduce wheat last, as people usually find it causes the most problems.

If you get a reaction to a grain, avoid eating it for a month or two before trying to reintroduce it again. Wait until your body settles down and symptoms subside before introducing another grain.

If your symptoms are severe, it's a good idea to give your body a complete rest for at least 2–3 months. It can take as long as six months, or even a year, for your body to get back to normal and learn to cope again with foods that were previously eliminated.

SENSITIVITIES AND ALLERGIES

There is a distinction between "food sensitivity" and "food allergy". We often find that severe menopausal symptoms are caused by food sensitivities, rather than an actual food allergy. A small number of women discover they have a permanent allergy to a particular food and soon realize they are better off avoiding that food altogether, rather than suffering unnecessarily. Which foods contain grains? To get an idea of how prevalent grains are in our foods, next time you're in the supermarket, have a closer look at some of the labels. You may be surprised by what you find.

Wheat The most obvious foods containing wheat include bread, cookies, cakes, pasta, cereals and pastries, as well as flour and other ingredients. Wheat is also often found in prepared sauces and soups, and processed foods such as sausages. If you are on a wheat-free diet, avoid gluten-free products too, as some of these still contain wheat. Wheat is sometimes disguised as modified starch, rusk and cereal filler.

Oats These are usually found in porridge, oat cookies, flapjacks and oat flakes.

Rye This is found in rye bread (which can also contain wheat), pumpernickel and rye crackers.

Barley This is often found in tinned or packet soups, as well as barley-based drinks.

COPE WITH CRAVINGS

Craving specific foods, particularly chocolate, is very common. It affects a staggering 75 percent of women in the UK, with 60 percent admitting that chocolate is their problem. These cravings can get worse around the time of the menopause and they're the reason many women put on weight.

Interestingly, there's often a physiological reason for cravings. The brain and nervous system require a constant supply of good nutrients in order to function normally, but our stressful lives mean that we don't always eat as healthily as we should. We skip meals or eat on the run. As a result, our blood-sugar levels drop and we start to crave a glucose fix to give us energy.

Then we grab the nearest sweet snack, which produces a temporary energy buzz. Before long we're craving something sweet again, and the cycle continues.

The trick is to know how to effectively break this cycle, which often develops into a real addiction. Just like an addiction to alcohol, drugs, smoking or other habits, this involves a period of withdrawal.

ASSESS YOUR FOOD CRAVINGS

Answer "yes" or "no" to the following questions:

- *Are you embarrassed about the amount of chocolate and cookies you consume?*
- *Do you graze on chocolate, cookies and crisps/potato chips throughout the day?*
- *Do you make impulse purchases of junk food?*
- *Do you take sugar in your tea or coffee?*
- *Do you drink more than three soft drinks per week?*
- *Do you routinely eat sweet food after meals or in the evening?*
- *Do you eat your children's chocolate or treats?*
- *Do you prefer chocolate to sex?*
- *Do you have a stash of comfort food?*
- *If you don't have chocolate at home, do you sometimes go out especially to buy some?*
- *Do you eat cookies, cakes, fruit pies, desserts or other foods containing sugar most days?*
- *Do you eat more than three bars of chocolate per week?*
- *Do you regularly eat ice cream?*
- *Do you crave salty foods such as crisps/potato chips salted nuts, savoury spreads or soy sauce?*
- *Do you feel hooked on certain types of food?*
- *Have you ever eaten chocolate and hidden the wrappers so that no one else knows?*

If you answered "yes" to three or more of these questions, you need to take some action. Five "yes" ticks means things are out of your control, and over six means you're addicted to junk food! But there is a solution, so don't panic.

OVERHAUL YOUR DIET

When it comes to controlling your cravings, it's important to monitor what you eat and when you eat it. You'll be amazed how giving your diet an overhaul and making a few tweaks can help to keep your blood glucose levels on an even keel, which means you're not always longing for your next sugar fix. As a result, any excess weight will drop off. Here are some goals to aim for:

• *Make sure you are getting enough of the right nutrients to keep your blood glucose at optimum levels. Essential nutrients for regulating blood sugar are the B vitamins (necessary for optimum function of the brain and the nervous system), magnesium (necessary for normal hormone function) and the trace element chromium. We are born with only 1.8g/^{1}/₁₆oz of the trace mineral chromium and it gets less as we age. Magnesium is the most common deficiency among women, and B vitamins are often in short supply. All of these important nutrients are necessary for normal blood glucose control helping to keep our cravings at bay. The B vitamins, magnesium and chromium can be sourced in food – eat whole grains, chilli, black pepper, chicken and peppers. But you may also want to consider taking a specially formulated nutritional supplement that acts as a short-term nutritional prop to regulate blood sugar levels. For example, a chromium supplement containing B vitamins and magnesium.*

• *Consume nutritious food – little and often – to keep blood sugar levels constant. Eat breakfast, lunch and dinner every day, with a wholesome mid-morning and mid-afternoon snack.*

• *Eat fresh, home-cooked, nutritious foods whenever possible.*

• *Eat foods that are intrinsically sweet, such as dried fruit, fresh fruit, nuts and seeds.*

• *Relax while you're eating and enjoy your food.*

• *Plan your meals and snacks in advance (bearing in mind that calorie requirements are increased by up to 500 calories per day during the premenstrual week for women).*

• *Always shop for food after you have eaten, not when you are hungry.*

• *Cut down on tea and coffee. In large amounts, they can cause an increase in the release of insulin. Large amounts of sugar consumed in tea or coffee can also contribute to an unstable blood glucose level. Try rooibos tea, or coffee substitutes.*

• *Reduce your intake of alcohol.*

REV UP YOUR SEX LIFE

Many women find that their desire for sex starts to wane during the menopausal years and beyond. A study presented to the seventh European Congress on the menopause in Istanbul in 2006 revealed that 75 percent of British women feel their sex drive has reduced since the menopause.

Tiredness, lack of energy and mood swings can put a dampener on the most solid relationship. At the same time, falling levels of estrogen can result in the lining of your vagina becoming dry and uncomfortable. When the vaginal tissues dry out, penetration can become painful and, in extreme cases, can result in tearing and bleeding. If you are also suffering from night sweats, it's not surprising that you don't feel like having sex.

Many women suffer in silence, thinking sexual disinterest is an inevitable part of growing older. But the good news is it doesn't have to be this way. There are plenty of things you can do to naturally repair the vaginal lining, encourage the cells to produce mucus again and get your libido back.

ASSESS YOUR SEX DRIVE

Answer "yes" or "no" to the following questions:

• *Have you lost your sex drive?*
• *Do you have sex less often than you used to?*
• *Do you find sex painful?*
• *Does your vagina feel dry?*
• *Have you stopped looking forward to sex?*
• *Have you stopped communicating with your lover on an intimate level?*
• *Are you too tired for sex?*
• *Has your enjoyment of sex diminished?*
• *Do you make excuses in order to avoid having sex?*

If you answered "yes" to more than two of these questions, try the following measures to give your sex life a boost.

CORRECT YOUR DIET

In a study we carried out at the NHAS, 50 percent of women said they couldn't have an orgasm, 55 percent reported problems with vaginal dryness, 36 percent suffered from painful intercourse and 47 percent admitted a lack of sexual sensations. Our experience at the NHAS suggests these problems are probably related to underlying nutritional deficiencies that prevent the brain chemistry from working properly. This has a knock-on effect on sex hormone function.

Our research shows it is important to correct nutritional deficiencies and consume a nutrient-dense, isoflavone-rich diet to help put yourself on a more even keel emotionally. Follow the dietary guidelines outlined in the Natural Menopause Plan diet (see page 26) and try the recipes in Part 2 (see page 62).

TAKE SUPPLEMENTS

There are several specific supplements that have been shown in clinical trials to help boost libido and repair dry vaginal tissue. These include omega-7 (sea buckthorn oil), horny goat weed, ArginMax, St. John's wort and Arkopharma Phyto Soya Vaginal Gel, which can be applied directly to the vagina (see page 158). If you suffer from vaginal dryness, use a lubricant such as Yes organic gel when you have sex.

STAY PHYSICALLY IN TOUCH

If penetration is really painful, explore other avenues of giving each other pleasure. Go back to your courting days and indulge in plenty of kissing, cuddling and foreplay. The important thing is that you continue to communicate physically and emotionally – even if you don't have sex, you can keep a sense of sexual and sensual connection alive.

Try treating each other to a sensual massage using massage oil. Turn on some relaxing music, dim the lights and start stroking and caressing each other. Burning essential oils, such as jasmine, rose, ylang ylang, clary sage or sandalwood, may heighten your enjoyment.

TALK TO EACH OTHER

Expecting your partner to understand what is going on, without you explaining, is an easy trap to fall into and can quickly put a distance between you. Try to spend some time together to explain what you are going through. Ask for your partner's support.

TAKE FLOWER REMEDIES

If your relationship is less than healthy, a dose of flower remedies may help to bring back that loving feeling. Wild rose remedy is believed to renew interest in life and boost vitality, while olive is thought to have revitalizing properties. Larch can help if you have lost confidence in your ability to make love.

BOOST YOUR BRAIN POWER

Do you lose your train of thought, forget where you left your keys or what you went upstairs for? We all start to forget things as we age, say the experts. When asked to memorize a list of 75 words read out five times, the average 18-year-old scores 54, a 45-year-old scores 47 and a 65-year-old scores just 37.

And the reason? No-one knows for sure, but it's thought most midlife memory problems are due to poor concentration, lack of motivation, tiredness, anxiety or stress, rather than loss of brain cells. Feeling fuzzy-headed is also thought to be related to the hormonal ups and downs of the menopause.

As we grow older, our circulation slows down and less oxygen reaches our brain, so it's no surprise we aren't as sharp. Also, many of us don't stretch our brains as much as we could. Like muscles, our brain needs to be used to function at optimum levels.

ASSESS HOW SHARP YOU ARE

Answer "yes" or "no" to the following questions:
- *Do you ever forget what you went upstairs for?*
- *Can you remember telephone numbers?*
- *Do you find it hard to concentrate?*
- *Do you forget a person's name the moment after you've been introduced?*
- *Are you prone to absent-minded acts, such as putting milk in the cupboard?*
- *Have you ever missed an appointment because you forgot it?*
- *Do you have to write arrangements down the minute you make them for fear of forgetting them?*
- *Have you ever forgotten the name of someone you know well?*
- *Do you frequently lose your car keys?*
- *Have you ever forgotten what you were saying mid-sentence?*
- *Have you ever been about to mention something important, but gone completely blank?*
- *Have you ever put something in the oven and forgotten to take it out?*
- *Have you ever said you would do something for someone, but completely forgotten to do it?*

If you answered "yes" to more than three questions, try making the following changes.

GET THE RIGHT NUTRIENTS

In general, a healthy diet, regular exercise, not smoking and watching what you drink will help to keep your brain sharp and reduce your risk of dementia. There are also some specific nutrients that the brain depends on for good health. Foods rich in the antioxidant vitamins A, C and E help to mop up free radicals, the rogue molecules that can cause excessive cell damage in the body, including the brain. Good sources include richly coloured fruit and vegetables, such as bananas, red peppers, spinach and oranges.

Oily fish is rich in omega-3 fatty acids, as well as folic acid, all of which are vital for the smooth functioning of the brain and nervous system. Good sources include sardines, salmon, herring, pilchards and mackerel.

Research shows that eating soy improves memory not just in the younger generation but also in menopausal women. The estrogen-like effects of isoflavones have led to speculation that soy may also help to maintain cognitive function in older women and reduce the risk of Alzheimer's disease.

Several B vitamins are also essential for normal memory and mental performance. Zinc and magnesium are necessary for neurotransmitter metabolism in the brain.

You may also like to try taking a daily ginkgo biloba supplement. Ginkgo biloba is made from the leaves of the Chinese maidenhair tree and has gained recognition over the past 30 years as a brain tonic. It improves circulation, which in turn increases blood flow, carrying more nutrients and oxygen to the brain. This helps to restore short-term and long-term memory.

KEEP YOUR MIND ACTIVE

Many studies show that mental stimulation is the key to a good memory. The more active your brain is, the better your memory is likely to be. And the more different ways in which you use your mind, the easier you'll find it to remember things. It's all to do with being active, rather than passive: whether you actively concentrate and focus on things or whether you just let them wash over you. Try the following to sharpen your mental faculties:

- *Do a mental exercise such as a crossword or Sudoko puzzle every day.*
- *When working out your finances, ditch the calculator and use your brain instead.*
- *Take up new activities – gardening, knitting or anything else that is active and involves hand–eye or foot–eye coordination.*
- *Memorize your shopping lists.*
- *Stretch yourself with a game of chess or bridge.*
- *Work for as long as you can, keep up with your friends and join local social groups. Studies have shown that people who have plenty of friends, especially at work, do significantly better in memory and concentration tests than those who don't.*

BEAT STRESS AND DEPRESSION

Life without challenges would be very dull, and some stress can keep you on your toes. But too much stress is damaging, especially at this time of life, when you're being pulled in many directions. The pressure of balancing children, family, relationships, work and finances can take their toll. Women also become more vulnerable to negative thinking or depression in midlife. While some women are delighted to be done with having periods, others mourn the loss of their reproductive years. Plus it's common to have low levels of important nutrients at midlife and this can result in mood changes and low energy levels.

ASSESS YOUR MOOD AND STRESS LEVELS

Answer "yes" or "no" to the following questions:

• *Are you tired all the time?*

• *Do you have trouble sleeping or wake up in the middle of the night?*

• *Do you crave sugary foods?*

• *Do you keep bursting into tears?*

• *Do you get frequent headaches?*

• *Do you find it hard to make up your mind?*

• *Do you get butterflies in your stomach?*

• *Do you feel anxious or on edge for no special reason?*

• *Have you got emotional problems?*

• *Are your family relationships strained?*

• *Are you forgetful?*

• *Is your digestive system upset?*

• *Is your appetite reduced?*

• *Do you sometimes feel it's all too much?*

• *Do you find it difficult to communicate with people?*

• *Do you have too little time for yourself?*

• *Do you tend to dwell on your failures, rather than on your achievements?*

• *Are you unhappy with what you have achieved in life?*

• *Do you sometimes doubt your ability to succeed?*

• *Do you see life as all downhill from now on?*

• *Do you wish you were young again?*

If you have more than three "yes" answers, take action now to beat stress and improve your mood.

CREATE SOME "ME" TIME

Work out your priorities so that you can efficiently use your time and energy. Make a realistic "to do" list at the beginning of each day. Learn to say "no" to people. Spend your free time doing something relaxing that you enjoy: meditation, soaking in the bath, listening to your favourite music, going for a walk or reading a book. It's also important to work out what your priorities and values are at this time of life. Spend time getting to know yourself again, as well as time to laugh and share friendships. Team up with a friend who is also going through the menopause and offer each other help and encouragement.

EAT WELL AND STAY ACTIVE

Resist the temptation of comfort foods, such as chocolate, cakes, cookies, soft drinks and coffee. These interfere with your ability to absorb vitamins and minerals, often making you feel even worse. Eating fresh or dried fruit, nuts and seeds is a much healthier option. Include plenty of magnesium-rich foods in your diet, such as spinach, Brazil nuts and walnuts. Magnesium supports the nervous system and has calming properties, helping to tackle the tiredness caused by stress. Take a strong multivitamin and mineral supplement, such as Fema 45+, Gynovite or Blackmores Proactive Multi 50+, together with the herbs valerian (see page 38) and rhodiola, which help calm you down.

One of the best stress- and depression-busters is physical exercise (see page 50). Regular activity helps to speed up the metabolism and encourages the release of endorphins, the body's own feel-good hormones.

THINK POSITIVELY

The first step to changing the way you think is to learn to love yourself for what you are and to accept the stage of life you are in – to embrace midlife, not run away from it. View change as a natural, inevitable and exciting move forward, not a threat. This allows you to cope with whatever changes come your way. Being optimistic about the future is more likely to bring results than thinking about how good things used to be. There's lots of evidence to show that those who see life as a "glass half-full", rather than a "glass half-empty", stand a better chance of feeling content and fulfilled. Try creative visualization (see page 41) to help you think positively.

It also helps to keep a note of your daily achievements, however small. Get yourself a notebook and write in it on a daily basis as you would with a diary. Read back over it each week and congratulate yourself on how well you are doing.

A key part of the Natural Menopause Plan is to include plenty of naturally occurring estrogens (phytoestrogens), known as isoflavones and lignans, in your diet. Foods such as soy and flaxseeds, which are rich in these substances, have been found to significantly reduce menopausal symptoms for many women who eat them on a daily basis.

Contrary to many people's expectations, eating a diet that's rich in foods such as soy isn't bland or boring. On the following pages is a wide selection of quick and easy recipes that are specially designed to include phytoestrogens. They're also brimming with vital nutrients, such as calcium, magnesium and essential fatty acids and are guaranteed to tempt your taste buds. You'll find delicious shake, smoothie and crêpe recipes for breakfast. Lunch and dinner choices include fresh salads, flavour-rich soups, risotto, bakes, curries, stir-fries and soufflé, with plenty of options for both vegetarians and meat-eaters. For dessert or between-meal snacks you can choose from cheesecake, fruit salad, brûlée, and bars, cakes and breads – all of which will count toward your daily phytoestrogen intake.

I've devised a number of menu plans (see pages 146–9) for you to follow during the first four weeks of your new phytoestrogen-rich diet. Once you become familiar with the foods you need to eat, start to make your own menu plans. Your aim from now on is to consume 100mg of phytoestrogens little and often over the course of each day (see page 27).

PART 2
The Natural Menopause Plan Recipes

BREAKFASTS

Rhubarb & Blueberry Smoothie

225g/8oz/1¾ cups rhubarb,
  trimmed and roughly chopped
3 tbsp honey
225g/8oz/1½ cups blueberries
500ml/17fl oz/2 cups chilled
  soy milk
¼ tsp vanilla extract
8 ice cubes, to serve (optional)

1 Preheat the oven to 200°C/400°F/Gas 6. Put the rhubarb on a baking sheet and drizzle with the honey. Roast for 15 minutes, or until tender, then set aside to cool.

2 Put the rhubarb and all the remaining ingredients in a blender or food processor and blend until smooth and creamy. Serve immediately with the ice cubes, if liked.

Banana Shake

2 very ripe bananas
25g/1oz/¼ cup ground almonds
¼ tsp ground nutmeg
500ml/17fl oz/2 cups chilled
  soy milk

1 Put all the ingredients in a blender or food processor and blend until smooth and creamy. Leave in the refrigerator for about 15 minutes, until chilled. Serve immediately.

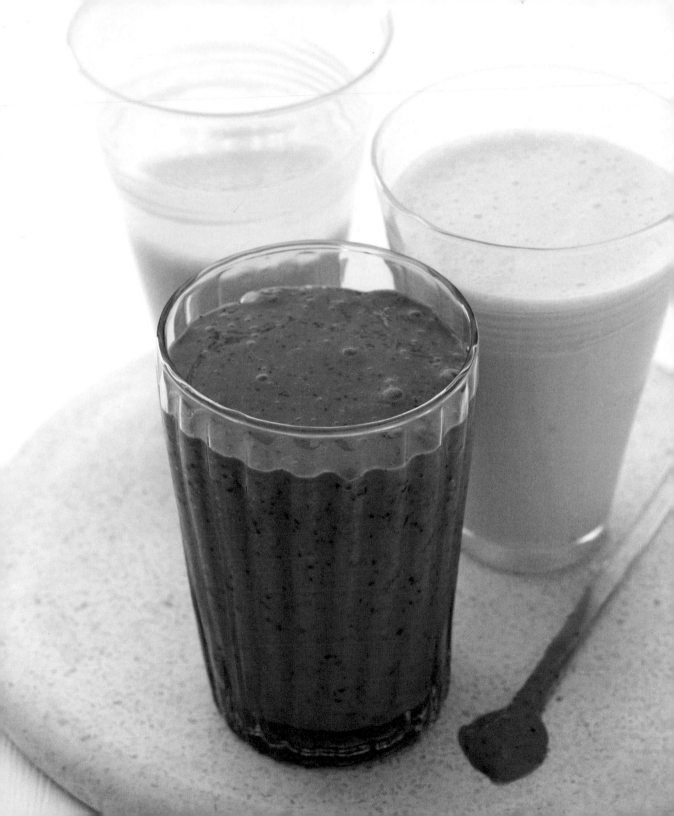

Honey & Cinnamon Soy Milk

500ml/17fl oz/2 cups chilled
   soy milk
1½ tbsp clear honey
¼ tsp cinnamon
8 ice cubes, to serve (optional)

1 Put all the ingredients in a blender or food processor and blend until light and frothy. Serve immediately, adding ice cubes if liked.

Creamy Banana & Date Shake

50g/1¾oz silken tofu
1 small, very ripe banana
4 dates, pitted
75ml/2½fl oz/⅓ cup apple juice
8 ice cubes, to serve (optional)

1 Put all the ingredients in a blender or food processor and blend until smooth and creamy. Serve immediately, adding ice cubes if liked.

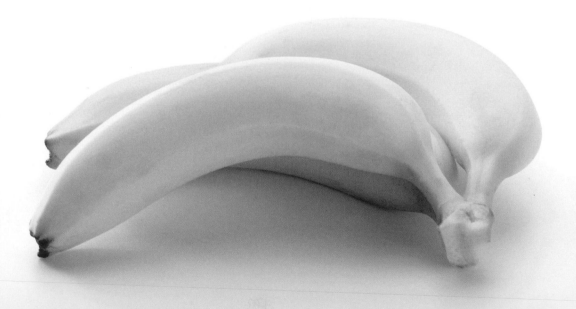

Fruit & Nut Shake

3 pieces of fruit, for example,
 1 mango, 1 pear and 1 apple,
 peeled, deseeded/cored
 and chopped
25g/1oz/¼ cup ground almonds or
 golden flaxseeds
500g/1lb 2oz/2 cups plain yogurt
8 ice cubes, to serve (optional)

1 Put all the ingredients in a blender or food processor and blend until smooth
 and creamy. Serve immediately, adding ice cubes if liked.

Scrambled Tofu

1 tbsp soy oil
1 small onion, finely chopped
1 carrot, finely chopped
1 potato, diced
570g/1lb 4½oz tofu, diced
1½ tsp turmeric
½ tsp black pepper
2 tomatoes, halved, to serve
4 mushrooms, to serve
4 slices of rye bread, toasted,
 to serve

1 Heat the oil in a large frying pan over a low heat. Add the onion and cook,
 stirring occasionally, for 2–3 minutes until it starts to turn golden.
2 Add the carrot and potato and cook, stirring frequently, for a further
 10 minutes, or until slightly soft. Stir in the tofu, turmeric and black pepper,
 cover with a lid and cook for 5 minutes, or until the mixture is heated through
 and has absorbed all the flavours.
3 Meanwhile, preheat the grill/broiler to medium. Grill/broil the tomatoes and
 mushrooms for 6–7 minutes, or until their tops are slightly golden.
4 Serve the scrambled tofu hot, with the tomatoes, mushrooms and
 rye bread.

Banana Oat Crêpes

50g/1¾oz/½ cup rolled oats
50g/1¾oz/heaped ½ cup soy flour
1 tbsp rice flour
1 tbsp baking powder
240ml/8fl oz/1 cup
   unsweetened soy milk
2 bananas, thinly sliced
1 tbsp sunflower oil
maple syrup, soy yogurt and
   fruit, to serve

1 Put the oats in a large mixing bowl and sift in the flours and baking powder. Make a well in the middle and pour in the soy milk, beating with a wooden spoon to form a smooth batter. Add the bananas and stir in gently until mixed together. Cover the mixture and leave to stand for at least 10 minutes or up to 30 minutes in the refrigerator.

2 Heat a large non-stick frying pan over a medium heat until hot. Add half the oil and tilt the pan so the oil covers the bottom completely. Pour 2 tablespoons of the batter into the pan and tilt the pan so the mixture covers the bottom. Cook for about 2 minutes until bubbles appear on the surface, then flip it over with a spatula. Cook for a further 1 minute, or until the bottom is slightly golden, then transfer to a plate.

3 Repeat with the remaining batter and oil, keeping the cooked crêpes warm. Serve warm with syrup, yogurt and fruit.

Soy & Buckwheat Crêpes

50g/1¾oz/heaped ⅓ cup
   buckwheat flour
50g/1¾oz/heaped ½ cup soy flour
½ tsp cinnamon
¼ tsp ground nutmeg
1 egg, beaten
300ml/10½fl oz/scant 1¼ cups
   unsweetened soy milk
2 tbsp soy oil
stewed fruit or sugar-free jam,
   to serve

1 Sift the flours and spices into a large mixing bowl and make a well in the middle. Add the egg, beating slowly with a wooden spoon to mix together. Pour in the soy milk and beat to form a smooth batter. Cover the batter and leave to stand for 10–30 minutes in the refrigerator.

2 Heat a large non-stick frying pan over a medium heat until hot. Add half the oil and tilt the pan so the oil covers the bottom completely. Spoon 2 tablespoons of the batter into the pan and tilt the pan so the mixture covers the bottom. Cook for 2 minutes, or until the underside is slightly golden, then flip it over with a spatula. Cook for a further 1 minute until the underside is slightly golden, then transfer to a plate.

3 Repeat with the remaining batter and oil, keeping the cooked crêpes warm. Serve warm with fruit or jam.

Soy & Rice Crêpes

50g/1¾oz/heaped ½ cup soy flour
50g/1¾oz/heaped ¼ cup rice flour
1 egg, beaten
300ml/10½fl oz/scant 1¼ cups
  unsweetened soy milk
2 tbsp soy oil
berries with honey or sugar-free
  jam, to serve

1 Sift the flours into a large mixing bowl and make a well in the middle. Add the egg, beating slowly with a wooden spoon to mix together. Pour in the soy milk and beat to form a smooth batter. Cover the batter and leave to stand for 10–30 minutes in the refrigerator.

2 Heat a large non-stick frying pan over a medium heat until hot. Add half the oil and tilt the pan so the oil covers the bottom completely. Spoon 2 tablespoons of the batter into the pan and tilt so the mixture covers the bottom. Cook for about 2 minutes until little bubbles appear and the crêpe is slightly golden, then flip it over with a spatula. Cook for a further 1 minute, or until the underside is slightly golden, then transfer to a plate.

3 Repeat with the remaining batter and oil, keeping the cooked crêpes warm. Serve warm with berries, and honey or jam.

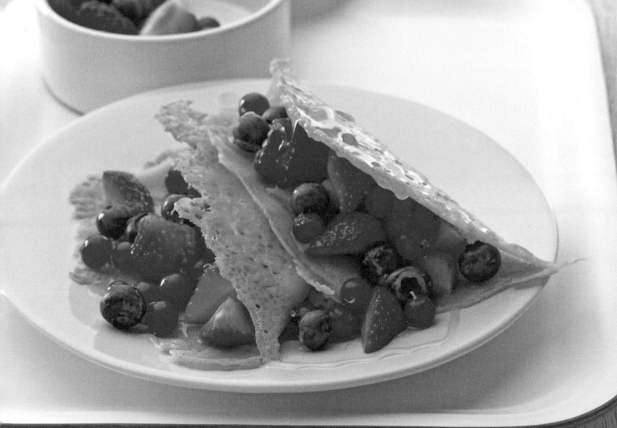

Crunchy Almond Granola

450g/1lb/4½ cups rolled oats
100g/3½oz/⅔ cup sunflower seeds
225g/8oz/1⅓ cups chopped
   almonds
150ml/5fl oz/scant ⅔ cup brown
   rice malt
150ml/5fl oz/scant ⅔ cup soy oil
150ml/5fl oz/scant ⅔ cup apple
   juice
225g/8oz/scant 2 cups
   raisins
100g/3½oz/heaped 1 cup
   desiccated/dried shredded
   coconut
soy milk or soy yogurt,
   to serve

1 Preheat the oven to 150°C/300°F/Gas 2. Mix together the oats, sunflower seeds and almonds in a large mixing bowl. Whisk the rice malt, oil and apple juice together in a jug and pour it over the mixture. Spread the mixture evenly onto a baking sheet and bake for 35 minutes, or until light brown, stirring every 5–10 minutes.

2 Remove from the oven and leave to cool, then return it to the mixing bowl. Stir in the raisins and desiccated/dried shredded coconut, mixing thoroughly. Serve with soy milk or soy yogurt. The remaining muesli can be stored in an airtight container for up to 4 weeks.

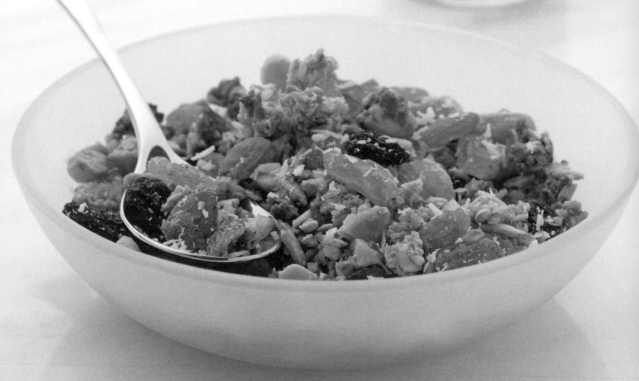

Phyto Sprinkle

60g/2¼oz/heaped ⅓ cup almonds
60g/2¼oz/½ cup sunflower seeds
60g/2¼oz/½ cup pumpkin seeds
60g/2¼oz/⅓ cup golden
   flaxseeds
cereal or fruit and natural yogurt,
   to serve

1 Put all the ingredients in a blender or food processor and pulse briefly
   until coarsely chopped.
2 Sprinkle over cereal or fruit and yogurt to serve. The remaining mixture
   can be stored in an airtight container for up to 4 weeks.

Phyto Muesli

375g/13oz/1¼ cups puffed rice
225g/8oz/8 cups cornflakes
100g/3½oz/⅔ cup chopped
   almonds
100g/3½oz/½ cup pumpkin seeds
100g/3½oz/heaped ¾ cup
   chopped pecans
100g/3½oz/⅔ cup sesame seeds
100g/3½oz/⅔ cup pine nuts
90g/3¼oz/heaped ½ cup flaxseeds
140g/5oz/heaped 1 cup
   raisins
100g/3½oz/heaped ½ cup
   unsulphured dried apricots,
   chopped
soy yogurt or soy milk,
   and fruit, to serve

1 Mix all the ingredients together in a large mixing bowl.
2 Serve with soy yogurt or soy milk, and fruit. The remaining muesli can be
   stored in an airtight container for up to 4 weeks.

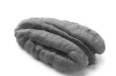
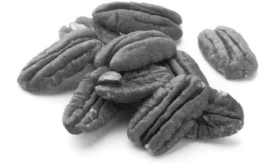

Porridge with Spiced Fruit Compôte

180g/6½oz/1¾ cups rolled oats
1l/35fl oz/4 cups soy milk
salt
plain yogurt, to serve

COMPÔTE
100g/3½oz/scant ½ cup caster/
    superfine sugar
150g/5½oz/scant 1 cup dried figs,
    chopped
100g/3½oz/heaped ½ cup
    unsulphured dried apricots,
    chopped
3 tbsp dried cranberries
2 cinnamon sticks
4 cloves
juice of 1 lemon, plus 2 strips
    of zest

1 To make the compôte, pour 250ml/9fl oz/1 cup water into a medium-size saucepan and add the sugar, dried fruit, cinnamon sticks, cloves and lemon zest. Bring to the boil over a medium heat, then reduce the heat to low and simmer for about 10 minutes, or until the fruit is soft and plump and the liquid has evaporated.

2 Add the lemon juice to the pan. Remove the pan from the heat and set aside for 2 minutes to cool slightly.

3 Put the oats and soy milk in a medium-size saucepan. Season lightly with salt and bring to the boil, then reduce the heat to low and simmer for about 10 minutes, stirring continuously until the porridge is thick and creamy. Serve hot with the fruit compôte and yogurt.

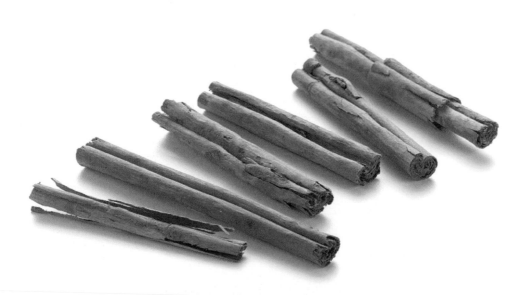

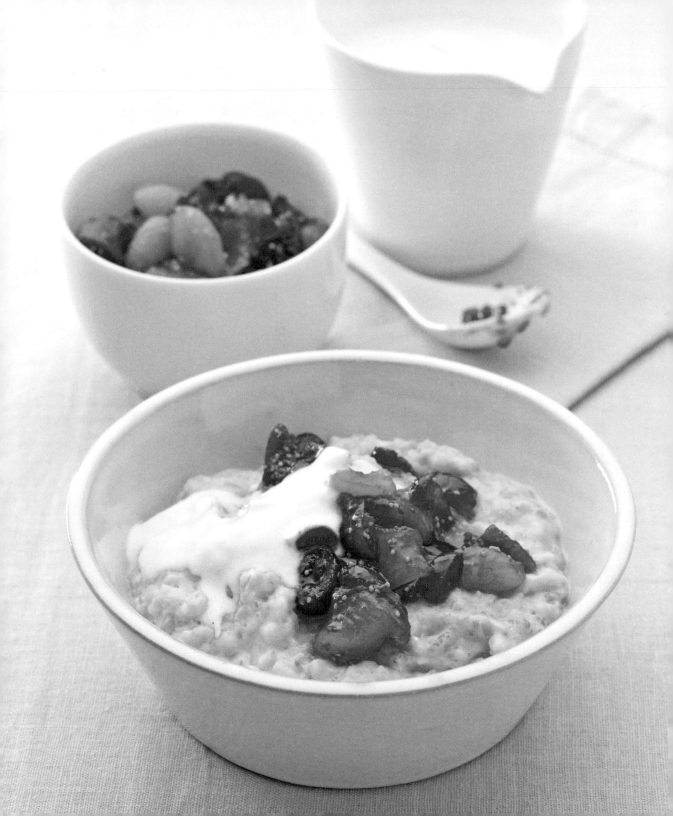

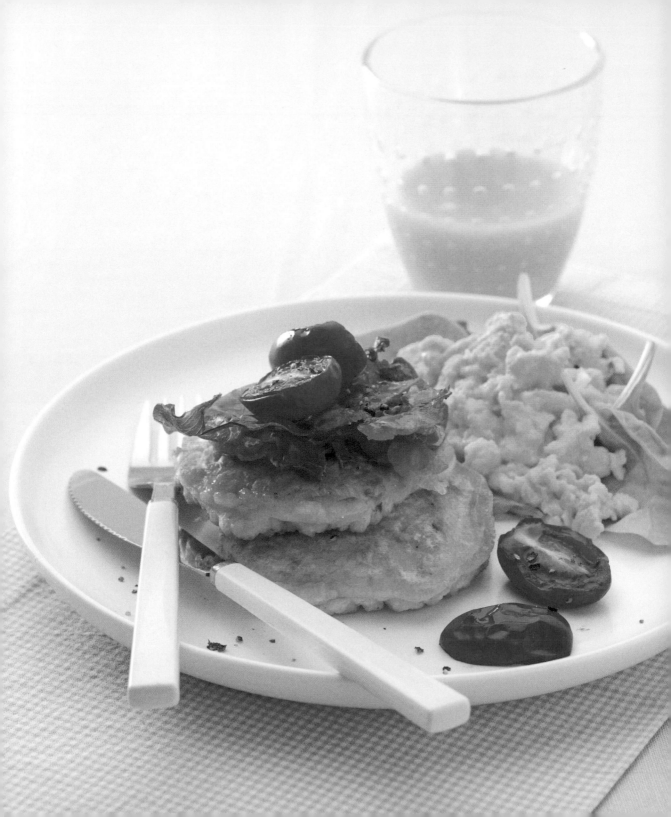

Chilli & Corn Fritters with Scrambled Eggs

150g/5½oz/1¼ cups plain/
  all-purpose flour
1 tsp baking powder
2 eggs, beaten
125ml/4floz/½ cup unsweetened
  soy milk
200g/7oz/1 cup canned
  sweetcorn/corn kernels,
  drained and rinsed
1 small red chilli, finely chopped
2 tbsp vegetable oil
8 baby plum tomatoes, halved
6 slices of prosciutto
salt and freshly ground black
  pepper
baby spinach leaves, to serve

SCRAMBLED EGGS
4 eggs
60ml/2fl oz/¼ cup unsweetened
  soy milk
30g/1oz/2 tbsp butter
freshly ground black pepper

1 Sift the flour and baking powder into a large mixing bowl and make a well in the middle. Add the eggs, beating slowly with a wooden spoon to mix together. Pour in the soy milk and add the sweetcorn/corn kernels and chilli. Season lightly with salt and pepper and beat to form a smooth batter. Cover the batter and leave to stand for 10–30 minutes in the refrigerator.

2 Heat a large non-stick frying pan over a medium heat until hot. Add half the oil and tilt the pan so the oil covers the bottom completely. Spoon 2 tablespoons of the batter into the pan and cook for 2 minutes, or until golden brown, then flip it over with a spatula. Cook for a further 2 minutes until golden brown and cooked through. Remove from the pan, drain on kitchen paper and keep warm. Repeat with the remaining batter and oil.

3 Meanwhile, preheat the grill/broiler to medium. Grill/broil the tomatoes and prosciutto for 2 minutes, or until the prosciutto turns slightly golden.

4 To make the scrambled eggs, beat the eggs in a small mixing bowl. Stir in the soy milk and season lightly with pepper. Melt the butter in a non-stick frying pan over a low heat. Pour in the egg mixture and cook gently, stirring frequently, for a few minutes until the mixture sets.

5 Serve the warm fritters topped with the grilled/broiled prosciutto and tomatoes, alongside the scrambled eggs on a bed of spinach leaves.

LUNCHES

Brown Rice & Watercress Salad

175g/6oz/scant 1 cup long-grain brown rice
1 bunch of watercress, roughly chopped
100g/3½oz/½ cup canned sweetcorn/ corn kernels, drained and rinsed
1 green pepper, deseeded and chopped
freshly ground black pepper
salad dressing, to serve

1 Put the rice in a saucepan and cover with 500ml/17fl oz/2 cups cold water. Bring to the boil over a high heat, then reduce the heat to medium and simmer for 25 minutes, or until the rice is tender and the water has been absorbed. Transfer the rice to a serving bowl and leave to cool.

2 Put the remaining ingredients into the serving bowl, season with black pepper and mix together. Serve with salad dressing.

Pictured right

Sweet Potato Salad

450g/1lb sweet potatoes, peeled and cubed
1–2 garlic cloves, crushed
1 tbsp chopped parsley leaves
1 tbsp chopped basil leaves
1 tbsp chopped chives
2 spring onions, chopped
1 tbsp soy oil
juice of 1 lemon
freshly ground black pepper

1 Put the sweet potatoes in a steamer and steam over a high heat for 10 minutes, or until cooked. Transfer them to a serving bowl and leave to cool.

2 Put the remaining ingredients in the serving bowl, season with black pepper, mix together and serve.

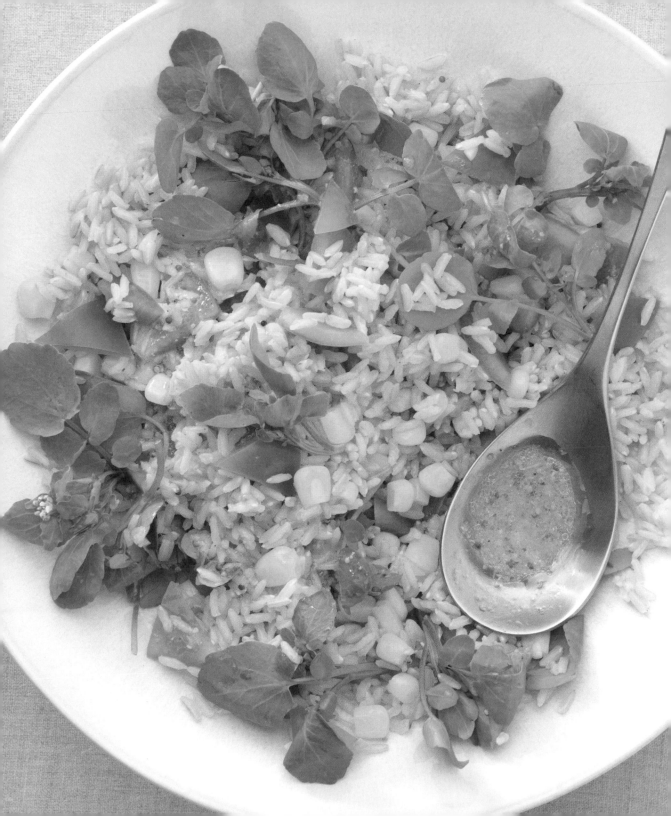

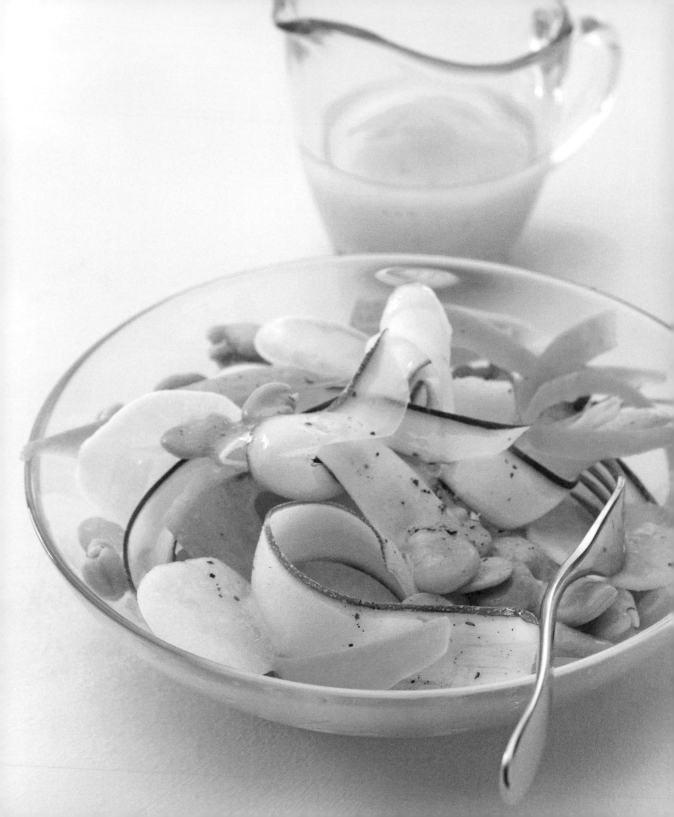

Oriental Rice Salad

50g/1¾oz/¼ cup long-grain white or brown rice
150g/5½oz/¾ cup basmati rice
1 tbsp sunflower oil
6 spring onions/scallions, finely chopped
1 red pepper, deseeded and thinly sliced lengthways
1 yellow pepper, deseeded and thinly sliced lengthways
50g/2oz mangetout/snow peas
100g/4oz/heaped 1 cup bean sprouts
2 tbsp tamari or soy sauce
1 tbsp lemon juice
100g/4oz/heaped ⅓ cup sprouted mung beans
freshly ground black pepper

1 Put both types of rice in a saucepan and cover with boiling water. Cook over a medium heat for 12–15 minutes until tender. Drain, rinse with boiling water, then drain again and set aside.

2 Heat the oil in a frying pan over a medium heat and add the spring onions/scallions, peppers, mangetout/snow peas and bean sprouts. Fry for a few minutes, stirring occasionally, until just tender and light brown.

3 Add the tamari, lemon juice, mung beans and the cooked rice and season with black pepper. Continue to fry, stirring continuously, until all the grains are evenly coated. Serve either hot or cold.

VARIATION *For a more substantial salad, add tofu, chicken or prawns/shrimp.*

Summer Salad

225g/8oz/1¼ cups shelled broad/fava beans
2 courgettes/zucchini, cut into ribbons
4 carrots, peeled and cut into ribbons
4 baby turnips, peeled and cut into ribbons
55g/2oz baby spinach
freshly ground black pepper
salad dressing, to serve

1 Put the broad/fava beans in a steamer and steam over a high heat for 5 minutes, or until lightly cooked. Transfer to a serving bowl and leave to cool completely.

2 Put the remaining ingredients in the serving bowl, mix together and serve with salad dressing.

Pictured left

Niçoise Salad with Soy Dressing

3 eggs
8 small potatoes, halved
4 tuna steaks
olive oil, for brushing
200g/7oz fine/thin green beans
10 cherry tomatoes, halved
100g /3½oz/¾ cup black olives
1 baby cos/romaine lettuce, leaves
  roughly torn

DRESSING
150g/5½oz silken tofu
100ml/3½fl oz/scant ½ cup
  unsweetened soy milk
1 garlic clove, chopped
1 tsp Dijon mustard
2 tbsp lime juice
freshly ground black pepper

1 Put the eggs in a small saucepan and cover with cold water. Bring to the boil over a high heat, then reduce the heat to low and simmer for 5 minutes. Remove the pan from the heat, drain the water from the pan and then leave the eggs to stand under cold running water for 1 minute. Leave the eggs in the pan of cold water for a further 2 minutes, then peel and set aside.

2 Put the potatoes in a saucepan and cover with cold water. Bring to the boil over a high heat, then reduce the heat to medium and simmer for 10 minutes, or until just tender. Drain and leave to cool.

3 Preheat the grill/broiler to high. Brush the tuna steaks lightly with oil and grill/broil for 2–3 minutes on each side until brown on the outside and slightly pink in the middle. Break the tuna into bite-size pieces with a fork.

4 Put the beans in a steamer and steam for 5 minutes. Remove the steamer from the heat and rinse the beans under cold running water, drain well and transfer to a large salad bowl.

5 Cut the eggs in half and add them to the beans. Add the potatoes, tuna, tomatoes, olives and lettuce and toss together gently.

6 Put all the ingredients for the dressing in a blender or food processor and blend until smooth. Season lightly with pepper, drizzle the dressing over the salad and serve.

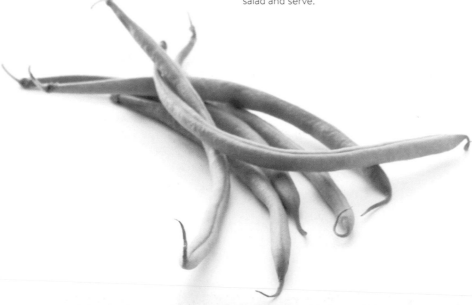

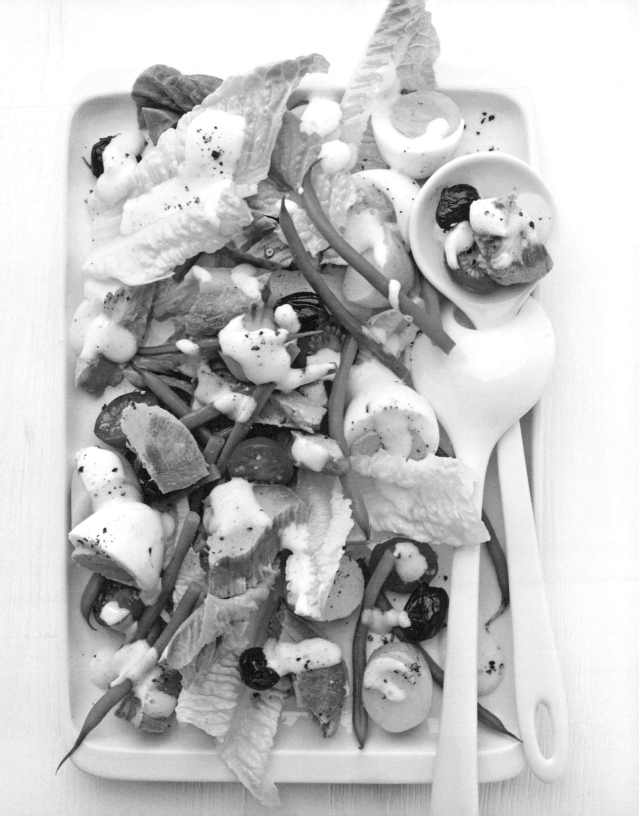

Apple & Nut Salad

4 red apples, peeled, quartered
  and cored
juice of ½ lemon
½ cucumber, cut into batons
6 celery sticks, chopped
1 bunch of spring onions/scallions,
  sliced
75g/2½oz/½ cup unroasted,
  salt-free peanuts
salad dressing, to serve

1 Cut each of the apple quarters into 3 slices and dip into the lemon juice to avoid discolouration.
2 Put the apple slices into a serving bowl, add the remaining ingredients, mix together and serve with salad dressing.

Endive, Fruit & Nut Salad

2 heads of curly endive/chicory
  lettuce, leaves torn into pieces
3 oranges
25g/1oz/¼ cup flaked/sliced almonds
25g/1oz/¼ cup walnuts, chopped
2 apples, cored and sliced into
  wedges
75g/2½oz seedless grapes
1 tbsp lemon juice

1 Put the endive/chicory leaves in a salad bowl.
2 Grate the zest of 1 orange into a large bowl. Peel the oranges, break the flesh into segments and put them in the bowl. Add the nuts, apples, grapes and lemon juice. Mix well and put on top of the endive/chicory.
3 Chill in the refrigerator for 10 minutes, then serve.

Coleslaw

1 white cabbage, cored and finely
  shredded
5 carrots, coarsely grated
1 large apple, coarsely grated
50g/1¾oz/scant ½ cup raisins
4 tbsp soy yogurt
4 tbsp soy mayonnaise
freshly ground black pepper

1 Put the cabbage, carrots, apple and raisins in a serving bowl.
2 Whisk together the soy yogurt and soy mayonnaise in a small jug and season with pepper. Pour over the salad, mix in well and serve.

Bean Salad

115g/4oz/½ cup dried kidney beans
115g/4oz/heaped ½ cup dried
   haricot/navy beans
115g/4oz/½ cup dried chickpeas
1 bay leaf
2 thyme sprigs
115g/4oz/scant ⅔ cup shelled
   broad/fava beans
1 garlic clove, crushed
2 tbsp extra virgin olive oil
2 tbsp finely chopped parsley
   leaves
1 onion, finely chopped
½ tsp ground cumin seeds

1 Put the kidney beans, haricot/navy beans and chickpeas in a bowl, cover with
   cold water and leave to soak overnight, or for at least 12 hours.
2 Drain the beans and chickpeas and rinse thoroughly. Put them in a
   saucepan, cover with cold water and bring to the boil over a high heat. Boil
   for 10 minutes, then reduce the heat to low and add the bay leaf and thyme.
   Cover with a lid and simmer for 1–1½ hours until tender. Drain the beans and
   leave to cool.
3 Put the broad/fava beans in a steamer and steam over a high heat for
   5 minutes, or until lightly cooked. Set aside and leave to cool.
4 Put the garlic in a serving bowl and pour in the oil. Add the beans, chickpeas,
   parsley, onion and cumin seeds. Mix together and serve.

Orange & Avocado Salad

2 avocados, peeled, pitted and
   chopped
4 tomatoes, sliced
4 oranges, peeled and separated
   into segments
2 spring onions/scallions, finely
   chopped
12 lettuce leaves

DRESSING
2 tbsp lemon juice
2 tbsp orange juice
2 tsp flaxseed oil
1cm/½in piece of root ginger,
   peeled and finely chopped

1 Put the avocados, tomatoes, oranges, spring onions/scallions and lettuce
   leaves in a serving bowl. Whisk together all the ingredients for the dressing in
   a jug and pour it over the salad. Mix together and serve.

Apple, Celery & Beetroot Salad

2 large beetroot/beets, peeled
   and sliced
2 apples, cored and sliced into
   wedges
2 celery stalks, diced
2 tbsp chopped walnuts

FRENCH DRESSING
1 tbsp Dijon mustard
1 tbsp clear honey
1 tbsp mayonnaise
4 tbsp extra virgin olive oil
2 tbsp white wine vinegar
freshly ground black pepper

1 Put the beetroot/beets in a steamer and steam over a medium heat for
   20 minutes, or until tender. Transfer them to a serving bowl and leave to cool.

2 Put the apple, celery and walnuts in the serving bowl and mix together.

3 To make the dressing, mix the mustard, honey and mayonnaise in a small
   mixing bowl. Mix the olive oil and vinegar in a separate jug. Slowly add the oil
   and vinegar to the mustard mixture, whisking all the time with a hand whisk
   until smooth. Pour the dressing over the salad, season with pepper and serve.

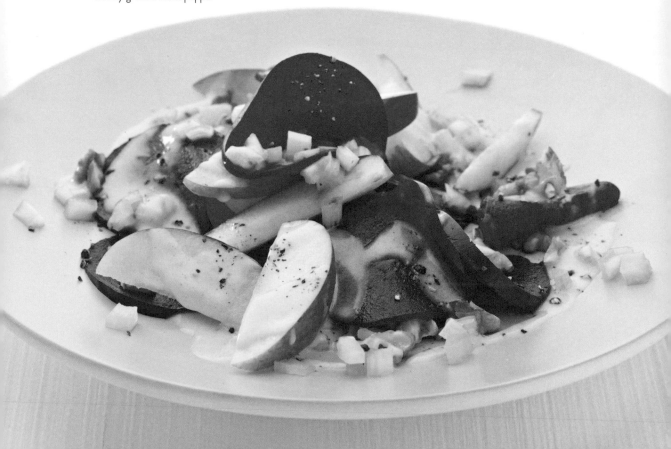

Lentil Scotch Eggs with Tofu Dressing

170g/6oz/scant 1 cup brown
   lentils, rinsed
4 eggs
1½ tbsp sunflower oil
2 large onions, finely chopped
1 garlic clove, crushed
1 tbsp oregano
1 tbsp basil
1 tbsp lemon juice
1 egg, beaten
1 tbsp sesame seeds
freshly ground black pepper
salad, to serve

DRESSING
100g/3½oz silken tofu
juice of 1 lemon
3 tbsp tahini
1 tsp tamari soy sauce
2 spring onions/scallions,
   finely chopped
1 tbsp finely chopped chives
1 tbsp finely chopped parsley
   leaves

1 Put the lentils in a saucepan and cover with cold water. Bring to the boil over a high heat, then reduce the heat to medium and simmer for 30 minutes, or until tender. Drain the lentils and set aside.

2 Put the eggs in a small saucepan and cover with cold water. Bring to the boil over a high heat, then reduce the heat to low and simmer for 5 minutes. Remove the pan from the heat, drain the water and then leave it to stand under cold running water for 1 minute. Leave the eggs in the pan of cold water for a further 2 minutes, then peel and set aside.

3 Preheat the oven to 180°C/350°F/Gas 4. Heat half of the oil in a frying pan over a medium heat and gently fry the onions for 6–8 minutes until soft and golden. Add the garlic, lentils, herbs and lemon juice. Season with black pepper. Mix well with a fork, adding a little of the beaten egg to bind if necessary.

4 Dip each boiled egg into the beaten egg and cover with one quarter of the lentil mixture. Brush again with beaten egg and roll in the sesame seeds. Cut 4 squares of foil, large enough to wrap each egg. Brush each of the eggs with the remaining oil, wrap with foil, put on a baking sheet and bake for 15 minutes.

5 To make the dressing, put the tofu, lemon juice, tahini and tamari in a blender or food processor. Blend until smooth and creamy, then stir in the spring onions/scallions, chives and parsley.

6 Remove the eggs from the oven and remove the foil carefully. Serve the eggs immediately with the tofu dressing and salad.

Parsnip & Apple Soup

1 tsp olive oil
1 onion, diced
6 large parsnips, peeled and
   roughly chopped
1 cooking apple, peeled, cored and
   roughly chopped
1.2l/40fl oz/4¾ cups vegetable
   stock
150ml/5fl oz/scant ⅔ cup skimmed
   milk
freshly ground black pepper

1 Heat the olive oil in a saucepan over a medium-low heat and fry the onion for about 3 minutes until translucent.
2 Put the parsnips and apple in the saucepan and add the stock. Bring to the boil over a medium heat, reduce the heat to low and cover with a lid. Simmer for 30 minutes, or until the parsnips are very soft.
3 Leave the soup to cool for 10 minutes, then transfer to a blender or food processor and blend until smooth.
4 Return the soup to the saucepan, add the milk and reheat gently over a low heat. Season with pepper and serve.

Watercress Soup

50g/1¾oz soy margarine
1 onion, finely chopped
6 potatoes, diced
1l/35fl oz/4 cups vegetable stock
a pinch of ground nutmeg
6 bunches of watercress, trimmed,
   plus extra to serve
freshly ground black pepper

1 Melt the margarine in a frying pan over a low heat, add the onion and fry gently for 5 minutes, or until the onion is transparent. Add the potatoes, stock and nutmeg, cover with a lid and simmer for 15 minutes, or until the potatoes are cooked. Add the watercress and simmer for a further 10 minutes, or until the ingredients have blended.
2 Leave the soup to cool for 10 minutes, then transfer to a blender or food processor and blend until smooth and creamy. Season with pepper and serve with a sprig of watercress.
Pictured right

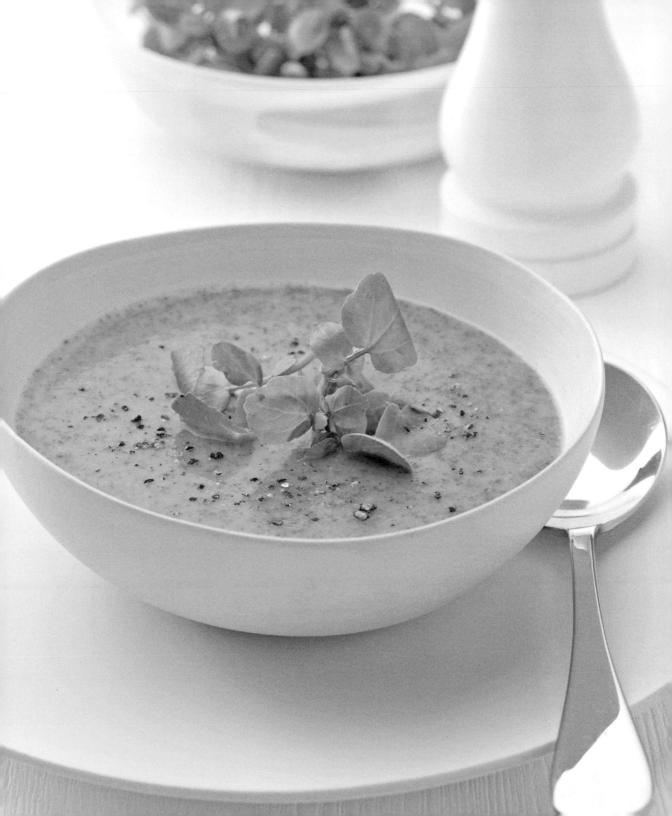

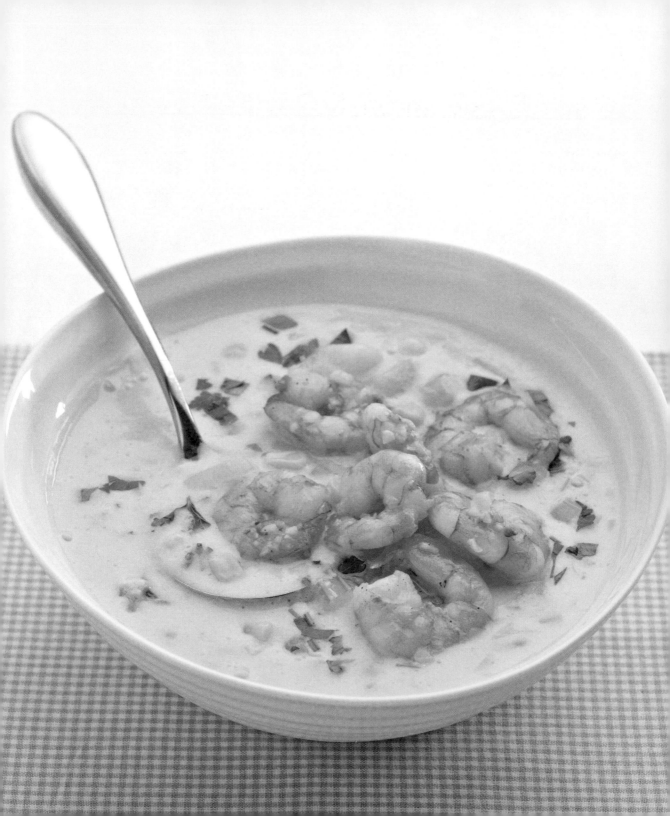

Corn Chowder with Garlic Prawns

2 tbsp olive oil
1 small onion, finely chopped
3 garlic cloves, finely chopped
1 potato, diced
200g/7oz/1 cup canned
   sweetcorn/corn kernels,
   drained and rinsed
1 celery stalk, diced
750ml/26fl oz/3 cups
   unsweetened soy milk
1 vegetable stock cube
250g/9oz peeled uncooked
   prawns/shrimp
4 handfuls flat-leaf parsley leaves,
   chopped
freshly ground black pepper

1 Heat 1 tablespoon of the olive oil in a saucepan over a medium heat. Add the onion and one-third of the garlic and cook for 3 minutes, or until the onion is translucent, stirring occasionally. Add the potato and cook for a further 2 minutes, or until the potatoes are heated through. Stir in the corn, celery and soy milk, and season with black pepper. Crumble in the stock cube and cover with a lid and bring to the boil over a high heat. Reduce the heat to low and simmer for 10 minutes, or until the vegetables are just tender.

2 Meanwhile, heat the remaining tablespoon of olive oil in a frying pan over a medium-high heat. Add the remaining garlic and the prawns/shrimp. Fry, stirring frequently, for 2 minutes, or until the prawns/shrimp turn pink.

3 Remove from the heat, add the parsley and stir thoroughly. Spoon the chowder into bowls and serve topped with the prawns/shrimp.

Pictured left

Chicken Noodle Soup

1l/35fl oz/4 cups chicken stock
1 garlic clove, finely chopped
2.5cm/1in piece of root ginger,
   peeled and grated
2 lemongrass sticks, finely
   chopped
2 skinless, boneless chicken
   breasts, cut into strips
250g/9oz shiitaki mushrooms
1 head of broccoli, cut into
   florets
250g/9oz soba noodles

1 Pour the stock into a large saucepan and add the garlic, ginger and lemongrass. Cover with a lid and bring to the boil over a medium heat. Reduce the heat to low, add the chicken and simmer for 8–10 minutes until the chicken is cooked through. Add the mushrooms and broccoli and simmer for a further 6 minutes, or until the broccoli is lightly cooked.

2 Put the noodles in a large saucepan and cover with boiling water. Cook over a medium heat until al dente, stirring occasionally, then drain, rinse with boiling water and drain again.

3 Divide the noodles into bowls, ladle the soup over them and serve.

Edamame Bean & Vegetable Soup

225g/8oz drained and
 rinsed, canned or frozen
 edamame beans
1l/35fl oz/4 cups vegetable stock
2 large carrots, grated
1 large parsnip, peeled and grated
2 leeks, finely sliced
1 small handful thyme, chopped
freshly ground black pepper

1 Rinse the edamame beans thoroughly and then drain. Put in a saucepan, pour over the stock and bring to the boil over a high heat. Reduce the heat to low, cover with a lid and simmer for 5 minutes, or until tender.

2 Put the mixture in a blender or food processor and blend until smooth. Pour back into the pan, add the carrots, parsnip and leeks and simmer for 10 minutes. Add the thyme and simmer for a further 5 minutes. Season with pepper and serve.

Mushroom & Mint Soup

4 large potatoes, chopped
1 small onion, chopped
900ml/31fl oz/scant 4 cups
 chicken stock
juice and zest of 1 lemon
1 tbsp chopped rosemary leaves
50g/1¾oz soy margarine
225g/8oz mushrooms, sliced
1 tbsp plain/all-purpose flour
2 tbsp finely chopped mint leaves
150ml/5fl oz/scant ⅔ cup
 unsweetened soy milk
freshly ground black pepper

1 Put the potatoes and onion in a large saucepan, add the stock, lemon juice and zest, and rosemary and season with pepper. Cover with a lid, bring to the boil over a high heat, then reduce the heat to low. Cover with a lid and simmer, stirring occasionally, for 25 minutes, or until the vegetables are tender. Leave to cool for 10 minutes, then transfer to a blender or food processor and blend until smooth.

2 Meanwhile, in a small saucepan, melt the margarine over a low heat. Add the mushrooms and stir until they are thoroughly coated in the margarine. Cook, stirring occasionally, for 10 minutes, or until the mushrooms are dark in colour. Sprinkle the flour over the mushrooms, stir gently until they are coated and then set aside.

3 Return the soup to the saucepan and add the mushrooms. Turn up the heat to medium and bring to the boil, stirring occasionally. Reduce the heat to low, stir in the mint and milk and cook for a further 5 minutes, or until the flavours have blended. Season with pepper and serve.

Hummus

225g/8oz/1 cup dried chickpeas
150g/5½oz/1 cup sesame seeds
2 tbsp tahini
2 tbsp soy oil
5 garlic cloves
juice of 3 lemons
a pinch of paprika (optional)
rice cakes, to serve

1 Put the chickpeas in a bowl, cover with cold water and leave to soak overnight, or for at least 12 hours.

2 Drain the chickpeas and rinse thoroughly. Put in a saucepan, cover with cold water and bring to the boil over a high heat. Boil for 10 minutes, then reduce the heat to low. Cover with a lid and simmer for 1–1½ hours until tender. Drain and leave to cool.

3 Put the sesame seeds, tahini, oil, garlic and half of the lemon juice in a blender or food processor and blend until smooth. Gradually add the chickpeas and remaining lemon juice, blending until smooth. Add a pinch of paprika for a touch of spiciness, if you like. Serve with rice cakes.

Carrot & Apricot Pâté

soy margarine, for greasing
75g/2½oz/scant ½ cup
   unsulphured dried apricots,
   finely chopped
75g/2½oz silken tofu
25g/1oz/¼ cup ground almonds
1 tbsp lemon juice
1 tsp ground cardamom
1 tsp ground nutmeg
250g/9oz carrot, grated
freshly ground black pepper
green salad and toast, to serve

1 Preheat the oven to 200°C/400°F/Gas 6 and grease a small loaf pan with soy margarine. Put the apricots in a saucepan and cover with 75ml/2½fl oz/ scant ⅓ cup water. Bring to the boil over a high heat, then reduce the heat to low and simmer for 10 minutes, or until soft.

2 Put the remaining ingredients in a bowl and mix together with a wooden spoon. Add the apricots and any remaining cooking liquid and mix thoroughly. Season with pepper.

3 Spoon the mixture into the loaf pan, cover with foil and bake for 45 minutes, or until firm to the touch.

4 Take the pan out of the oven and leave the pâté to cool completely. Chill the pâté in the refrigerator for 30 minutes, then remove from the pan, cut into slices and serve with salad and toast.

Tofu, Bean & Herb Stir-Fry

2 tbsp soy oil
250g/9oz tofu, cubed
2 garlic cloves, crushed
300g/10½oz green beans
3 tbsp mixed finely chopped
   herbs, such as thyme, parsley,
   chives or chervil
4 spring onions/scallions,
   thinly sliced
2 tbsp tamari soy sauce
freshly ground black pepper
rice or noodles, to serve

1 Heat 1 tablespoon of the oil in a frying pan or wok over a high heat until hot. Add the tofu and garlic and stir-fry for 2 minutes until the tofu absorbs the flavour of the garlic. Using a slotted spoon, remove the tofu and drain on kitchen paper.

2 Heat the remaining oil in the pan, add the green beans and fry over a medium heat for 4 minutes, or until the beans are lightly cooked. Add the herbs, spring onions/scallion and tamari and stir-fry for a further 1 minute.

3 Return the tofu to the pan and stir-fry for 1 minute until the flavours have merged. Season with pepper and serve immediately with rice or noodles.

Pictured right

Tempeh with Pak Choi & Noodles

450g/1lb tempeh, cut into
   2.5cm/1in cubes
200g/7oz egg noodles
1 tbsp olive oil
200g/7oz pak choi/bok choy,
   leaves separated

MARINADE
3 garlic cloves, finely chopped
2 onions, finely chopped
1 apple, peeled, quartered, cored
   and chopped
200ml/7floz/¾ cup sesame oil
200ml/7floz/¾ cup cider vinegar
juice of 2 lemons
60ml/2fl oz/¼ cup tamari soy
   sauce
2.5cm/1in piece of root ginger,
   peeled and sliced
2 tsp black peppercorns, crushed
12 cloves
1 cinnamon stick

1 Put the tempeh in an ovenproof dish. Mix together all the marinade ingredients in a large jug and pour the mixture over the tempeh. Cover with a lid and leave to marinate in the refrigerator for 6–8 hours, or overnight.

2 Preheat the oven to 190°C/375°F/Gas 5. Bake the marinated tempeh for 1 hour, or until golden and firm.

3 About 10 minutes before the tempeh finishes cooking, put the noodles in a large, heatproof bowl and cover with boiling water. Leave to stand for 5 minutes, then drain and rinse well.

4 Heat the olive oil in a wok over a high heat. Add the pak choi/bok choy and stir-fry for 2 minutes, or until the stalks are starting to soften. Stir in the noodles and fry for a further 1 minute.

5 Serve the pak choi/bok choy and noodles immediately with the tempeh.

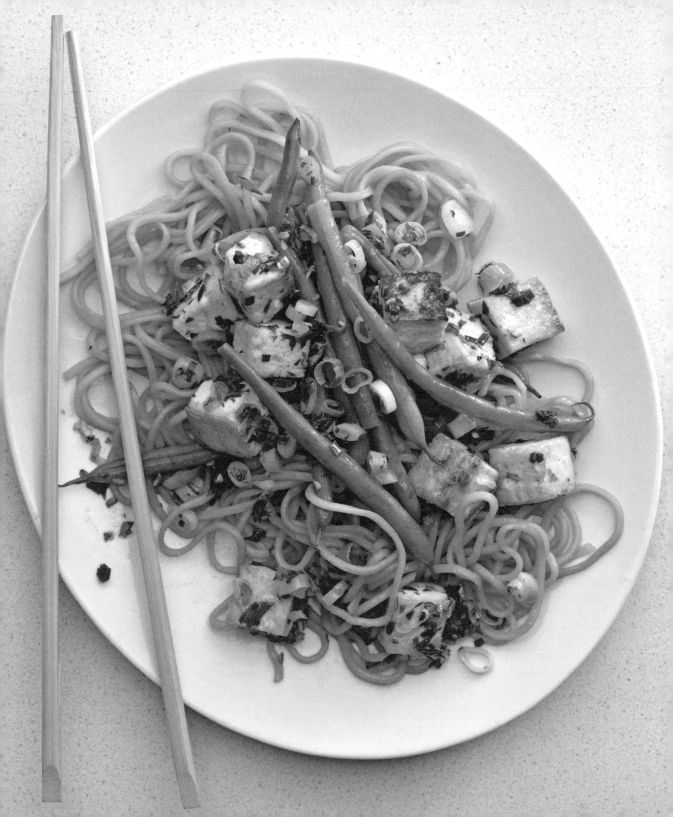

Turkish Tempeh on Pitta Bread

50g/1¾oz/¼ cup brown rice
2 tbsp soy oil
300g/10½oz tempeh, finely sliced
4 pitta breads, lightly toasted
110g/3¾oz/½ cup Hummus
  (see page 91)
2 tomatoes, diced
8 large lettuce leaves, shredded
115g/4oz/heaped ⅔ cup
  peanuts, finely chopped

1 Put the rice in a sieve/fine-mesh strainer and rinse thoroughly under cold running water. Put in a saucepan and cover with water. Bring to the boil and then turn down the heat to low and simmer, covered, for 25 minutes, or until tender. Drain and set aside, keeping the lid on to contain the heat.

2 Heat the oil in a frying pan over a medium heat, add the tempeh and fry for 2 minutes on each side, or until golden.

3 Spread each pitta bread with the hummus, then divide the tempeh over the top. Top with the rice, followed by the tomato, lettuce and peanuts. Serve warm.

Baked Potatoes with Spicy Soybeans

450g/1lb/2½ cups dried soybeans
3 bay leaves
4 large baking/Idaho potatoes,
  scrubbed and scored
2 tbsp soy oil
1 large onion, chopped
2 garlic cloves, chopped
5cm/2in piece of cinnamon stick
185ml/6fl oz/¾ cup passata
150ml/5fl oz/scant ⅔ cup molasses
150ml/5flozl/scant ⅔ cup Dijon
  mustard
1l/35fl oz/4 cups vegetable stock
2 tbsp apple cider vinegar
1 tbsp tamari soy sauce

1 Wash the beans and drain. Put in a large bowl, cover with cold water and leave to soak overnight, or for at least 12 hours.

2 Drain the beans and rinse thoroughly. Put them in a large saucepan, cover with cold water and bring to the boil over a high heat. Boil for 10 minutes, then reduce the heat to low. Add the bay leaves, cover with a lid and simmer for 2 hours, or until tender. Drain the beans and leave to cool.

3 Meanwhile, preheat the oven to 200°C/400°F/Gas 6. Bake the potatoes for 1 hour, or until tender.

4 Heat the oil in a saucepan over a medium heat and fry the onion and garlic for 3 minutes, or until the onions are translucent. Add the cinnamon and cook for 1 minute, stirring frequently. Stir in the passata, molasses, mustard, beans and stock and bring to the boil. Cover the pan, reduce the heat to low and simmer gently for 1 hour until the flavours have merged. Stir once during this time and add more stock if necessary.

5 Stir in the vinegar and tamari. Remove the cinnamon stick and serve the beans immediately, spooned over the potatoes.

Rosemary Arancini

500ml/17fl oz/2 cups
  unsweetened soy milk
500ml/17fl oz/2 cups chicken
  stock
40g/1½oz butter
1 onion, finely chopped
1 garlic clove, crushed
220g/7¾oz/1 cup risotto rice
60g/2¼oz mozzarella cheese, cut
  into 1cm/½in cubes
500ml/17fl oz/2 cups sunflower
  oil, for deep-frying
2 eggs, beaten
220g/7¾oz/2¼ cups dry
  breadcrumbs
12 small rosemary sprigs
salad, to serve

1 Pour the soy milk and stock into a saucepan over a medium heat and bring to
   the boil. Remove from the heat and set aside to cool for 5 minutes.
2 Heat the butter in large saucepan over a medium heat until hot. Fry the
   onion and garlic for 2–3 minutes, or until soft. Add the rice and stir for
   1 minute, or until the rice starts to turn clear. Reduce the heat to low, add a
   ladleful of the stock mixture and stir until the liquid is absorbed. Add more
   liquid gradually, stirring continuously until it is all absorbed. Remove the pan
   from the heat and leave to one side for 5 minutes for the risotto to cool.
3 Divide the risotto mixture into 12 pieces and roll each one into a ball. Gently
   press your thumb into each ball to make a hole, then put a cube of mozzarella
   inside. Pinch the rice mixture to enclose the cheese and roll again to make
   the surface smooth. Refrigerate the balls for 30 minutes.
4 Heat the oil in a frying pan over a medium heat until hot. Remove the rice
   balls from the refrigerator. Dip a ball first into the egg, then the breadcrumbs
   until evenly coated. Repeat with the remaining balls. Working in batches,
   spear each ball with a sprig of rosemary and deep-fry until golden brown.
   Using a slotted spoon, remove from the oil, drain on paper towels and keep
   warm. Serve warm with salad.

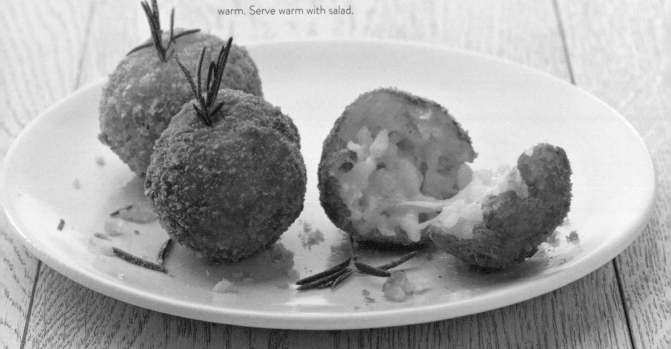

Potato Skins with Broccoli & Tofu Filling

4 large baking/Idaho potatoes,
   scrubbed and scored
225g/8oz broccoli, trimmed and
   cut into florets
1 tbsp sunflower oil
2 onions, finely chopped
100g/4oz mushrooms, chopped
¼ tsp ground nutmeg
285g/10oz tofu
1 handful of parsley, finely
   chopped
1 tbsp Dijon mustard
freshly ground black pepper
salad, to serve

1 Preheat the oven to 200°C/400°F/Gas 6. Put the potatoes on a baking sheet and bake for 1 hour, or until cooked through.

2 Put the broccoli in a steamer over a high heat and steam for 6 minutes until just tender but still bright green. Remove from the pan and set aside.

3 Heat the oil in a frying pan over a low heat and, stirring occasionally, fry the onion for 3 minutes, or until translucent. Add the mushrooms and continue to fry for a further 5 minutes, stirring often. Add the nutmeg, season with pepper and remove from the heat.

4 Slice the baked potatoes in half lengthways and scoop out the insides, leaving a thick shell of potato skin. Put the potato, steamed broccoli, tofu, parsley and mustard in a mixing bowl and mash together to make a smooth mixture. Add the mushrooms and onions and stir thoroughly. Spoon the mixture into the potato skins.

5 Return the potatoes to the oven for 15 minutes, or until warmed through. Serve immediately with salad.

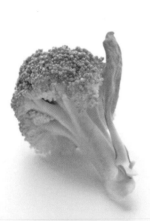
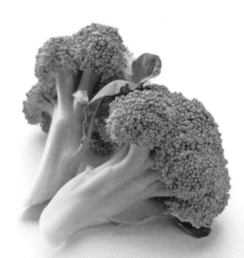

Refried Soybeans

450g/1lb/2½ cups dried
  soybeans
1 tbsp soy oil
1 onion, finely chopped
1 garlic clove, crushed
1 tsp sweet chilli sauce
rice, taco shells or baked
  potatoes, to serve

1 Put the soybeans in a large bowl, cover with cold water and leave to soak overnight, or for at least 12 hours.

2 Drain the beans and rinse thoroughly. Put the beans in a large saucepan, cover with cold water and bring to the boil over a high heat. Boil for 10 minutes, then reduce the heat to low. Cover with a lid and simmer for 2 hours, or until tender. Drain and set aside.

3 Heat the oil in a saucepan over a medium heat and fry the onion and garlic for 3 minutes, or until the onions are translucent. Stir in the soybeans and sweet chilli sauce and cook for 2 minutes, stirring continuously. Gently mash the mixture with a fork.

4 Serve warm with rice or taco shells or as a filling for baked potatoes.

Bean Burgers

100g/4oz/½ cup mixed dried
  beans, such as butter beans,
  soybeans or black-eyed beans
2 garlic cloves, crushed
1 onion, finely chopped
2 tomatoes, finely chopped
1 tsp black pepper
½ tsp chilli powder
1 tbsp sunflower oil
freshly ground black pepper
salad, to serve

1 Put the beans in a large bowl, cover with cold water and leave to soak overnight, or for at least 12 hours.

2 Drain the beans and rinse thoroughly. Put in a large saucepan, cover with cold water and bring to the boil over a high heat. Boil for 10 minutes, then reduce the heat to low. Cover with a lid and simmer for 1 hour, or until soft. Drain, mash well to make a thick paste and leave to cool.

3 Put the beans in a serving bowl and stir in the garlic, onion, tomatoes, pepper and chilli powder. Divide the mixture into 8 pieces and shape each piece into a ball with your hands. Flatten to form burgers.

4 Heat half the oil in a frying pan over a medium heat until hot. Add half the burgers and fry for 5 minutes on each side until browned. Keep warm while you cook the remaining burgers, adding the remaining oil as necessary. Serve with salad.

Bean Tacos

75g/2½oz soy mince/ground
  "meat" TVP
½ tsp Chinese five spice
2 tbsp soy yogurt
1 tbsp soy oil
1 onion, finely chopped
1 green pepper, deseeded and
  finely chopped
2 tbsp tomato purée/paste
400g/14oz canned mixed beans,
  such as kidney beans and black-
  eyed beans, drained and rinsed
8 taco shells
8 large lettuce leaves, shredded
4 tomatoes, diced
2 avocados, peeled, pitted
  and diced

1 Put the soy mince/TVP in a small heatproof bowl and pour in 125ml/
4fl oz/½ cup boiling water. Leave to stand for 10–15 minutes until the
water has been absorbed. Rinse and drain thoroughly.

2 Stir the five spice into the soy yogurt and set aside.

3 Heat the oil in a frying pan over a medium heat. Add the onion and pepper
and, stirring occasionally, fry for 3 minutes, or until tender. Add the tomato
purée/paste, mixed beans, soy mince/TVP and spicy yogurt mixture, and
pour in 60ml/2fl oz/¼ cup water. Cook for 6 minutes, or until the beans
have softened.

4 Remove the pan from the heat and spoon the bean mixture into the taco
shells, top with the lettuce, tomato and avocado, and serve.

Pictured right

Spanish Omelette

2 tbsp olive oil
3 small potatoes, sliced
1 red pepper, deseeded and cut
  into strips
1 red onion, halved and thinly
  sliced
2 rindless bacon slices, cut
  into strips
1 small handful of oregano leaves,
  finely chopped
6 eggs
125ml/4floz/½ cup unsweetened
  soy milk
freshly ground black pepper
salad, to serve

1 Heat the oil in a large, ovenproof, non-stick frying pan over a medium heat.
Add the potatoes and red pepper, cover with a lid and fry for 10 minutes, or
until the potatoes are cooked through, stirring occasionally. Add the onion
and bacon and cook for a further 10 minutes, or until the bacon is cooked
through, stirring frequently. Stir in the oregano and season with black pepper.

2 Preheat the grill/broiler to medium. Whisk together the eggs and soy milk
in a jug and pour it over the mixture in the pan. Cover again and cook over a
medium heat for 5 minutes, or until the bottom is golden and set.

3 Remove the pan from the heat and place under the grill/broiler for a further
10 minutes, or until the top is golden. Serve warm with salad.

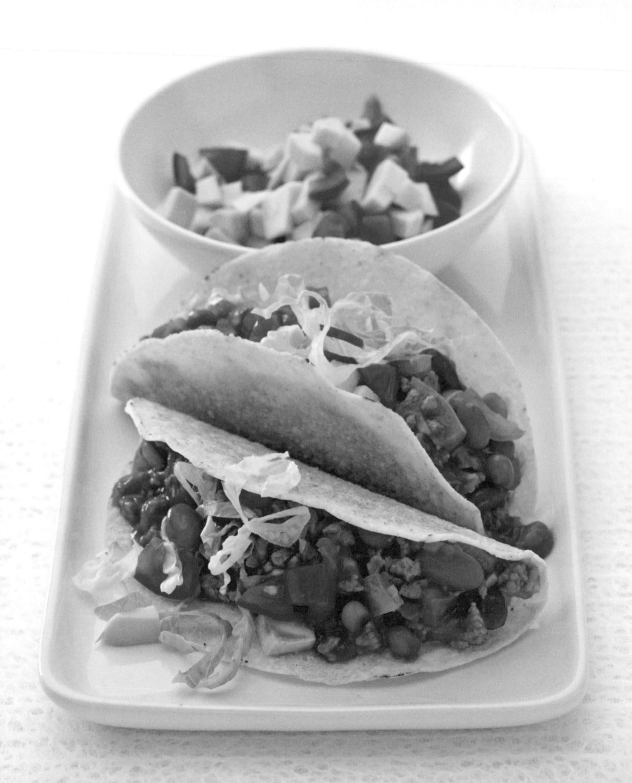

Lemon & Artichoke Risotto with Salmon & Asparagus

750ml/26fl oz/3 cups
 unsweetened soy milk
500ml/17fl oz/2 cups chicken
 stock
30g/1oz butter
1 tbsp olive oil, plus 1 tsp for
 rubbing
1 small red onion, thinly sliced
2 garlic cloves, finely chopped
½ preserved lemon, chopped
330g/11½oz/1½ cups risotto rice
290g/10¼oz marinated
 artichoke hearts, sliced
400g/14oz salmon fillets
1 bunch of asparagus, trimmed
freshly ground black pepper

1 Pour the soy milk and stock into a saucepan over a medium heat and bring to the boil. Turn the heat down to low, cover with a lid and simmer for 5 minutes.

2 Heat the butter and oil in a large saucepan over a medium heat until hot. Fry the onion and garlic for 2–3 minutes, or until soft. Add the lemon and rice and stir for 1–2 minutes, or until the rice starts to turn clear. Add a ladleful of the soy milk and stock mixture, reduce the heat to low and stir until all the liquid has been absorbed. Continue adding the liquid and stirring for about 20 minutes until it has all been absorbed. Add the artichokes, season with pepper and stir thoroughly.

3 Meanwhile, season the salmon with pepper and rub lightly with the oil. Cook the salmon in a frying pan over a medium heat for 2–3 minutes on each side until the flesh is cooked through. Transfer to a plate and flake into pieces with a fork.

4 Put the asparagus in a steamer and steam over a high heat for 5–6 minutes until cooked through. Remove from the pan and drain well.

5 Serve the risotto hot, topped with the salmon and asparagus.

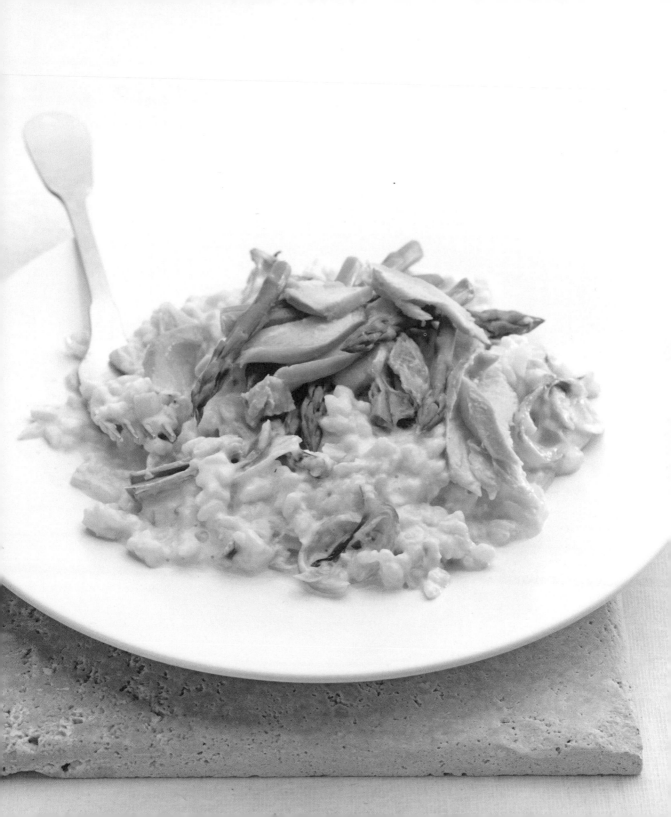

Mustard Cod Crêpes

350g/12oz cod fillets
50g/1¾oz sunflower margarine,
    plus extra for greasing
25g/1oz/scant ¼ cup plain/
    all-purpose flour
450ml/16fl oz/scant 2 cups
    unsweetened soy milk
juice of 1 lemon
2 tbsp Dijon mustard
freshly ground black pepper
lemon slices, to serve

CRÊPES
75g/2½oz/heaped ½ cup plain/
    all-purpose white flour
1 large egg, beaten
450ml/16fl oz/scant 2 cups
    unsweetened soy milk
2–3 tbsp sunflower oil

1 To make the filling, put the cod in a steamer and steam for 10–15 minutes, until the fish flakes easily and is cooked through. Using a fork, remove the skin from the fish and flake the flesh into small pieces.

2 Meanwhile, melt the margarine in a saucepan over a medium heat, stir in the flour and cook for 1 minute. Remove the pan from the heat and gradually stir in the milk until smooth and creamy. Return the pan to the heat and slowly bring to the boil, stirring continuously, until it resembles a blended sauce. Simmer slowly for about 3 minutes, stirring all the time, until it coats the back of a spoon. Stir in the lemon juice and mustard and season with black pepper. Remove the pan from the heat, spoon half of the sauce into a bowl and set aside. Stir the cod into the remaining sauce in the saucepan and set aside.

3 To make the crêpes, sift the flour into a large mixing bowl and make a well in the middle. Add the egg and half of the milk and beat slowly with a wooden spoon to incorporate the flour. Slowly beat in the remaining milk. Add a little extra milk if the batter seems thick.

4 Heat 1 teaspoon of the oil in a small frying pan over a high heat until hot. Pour in 3 tablespoons of the batter and tilt the pan so that the batter spreads evenly over the bottom. Cook for 2 minutes, or until golden brown underneath, then turn the crêpe over with a spatula and cook for a further 2 minutes, or until lightly golden.

5 Repeat with the remaining batter until you have made 12 crêpes. Pile one on top of the other with greaseproof/wax paper in between, and keep covered with a clean dish towel to keep warm until required.

6 Preheat the oven to 170°C/325°F/Gas 3 and grease an ovenproof dish with margarine. Spoon 2 tablespoons of the cod mixture onto one half of each crêpe and roll the crêpe over the mixture.

7 Put the crêpes in the dish and cover with the remaining sauce. Bake for 10 minutes, or until hot. Serve with the lemon slices on the side.

Haddock Baked in Foil

8 tomatoes

4 courgettes/zucchini, thinly sliced

6 celery stalks, sliced

1 red pepper, deseeded and cut
into strips

1 green pepper, deseeded and cut
into strips

150g/5½oz canned sweetcorn/
corn kernels, drained and rinsed

2 tbsp lemon juice

2 tbsp vegetable stock

4 haddock steaks

1 tbsp finely chopped parsley
leaves

freshly ground black pepper

broccoli and rice, to serve

1 Preheat the oven to 180°C/350°F/Gas 4. Cut a cross in the skins of the tomatoes with a sharp knife. Put in a large, heatproof bowl and cover with boiling water. Leave to stand for 2–3 minutes, then remove from the water, peel the skins and slice the flesh.

2 Put the tomato flesh and remaining vegetables in a saucepan and pour in the lemon juice and stock. Bring to the boil over a medium heat, reduce the heat, cover with a lid and simmer for 10 minutes, or until all the vegetables are cooked.

3 Put each piece of fish on a piece of foil large enough to wrap around it. Evenly divide the vegetables on top of the fish, sprinkle with the parsley and season with pepper. Wrap the foil over and secure the ends.

4 Bake for 30 minutes, or until the haddock is cooked through. Serve hot with broccoli and rice.

Poached Fish Balls

450g/1lb white fish fillets, skinned
and any remaining bones
removed

1 egg white

2 tsp cornflour/cornstarch

1 tsp vegetable oil

2 tbsp finely chopped coriander/
cilantro leaves

plain/all-purpose flour, for rolling

900ml/31fl oz/scant 4 cups
fish stock

freshly ground black pepper

vegetables or salad, to serve

1 Put the fish in a blender or food processor and blend until smooth. Add the egg white, cornflour/cornstarch, oil and coriander/cilantro and season with pepper. Blend again until thoroughly combined, then transfer to a bowl.

2 Using lightly floured hands, roll the mixture into 3cm/1¼in balls. Put on a lightly floured plate and chill in the refrigerator for 30 minutes.

3 Pour the fish stock into a large saucepan and bring to the boil over a medium heat. Reduce the heat to low, slip half of the fish balls into the stock and simmer for 5–6 minutes until cooked through. Remove from the stock with a slotted spoon, drain on paper towels and keep warm. Repeat with the remaining fish balls. Serve warm with vegetables, or serve cold with salad.

VARIATION *Instead of poaching the fish balls, flatten them gently with your hands and fry them in garlic-flavoured oil for 3 minutes on each side.*

Mackerel with Lemon & Ginger

4 mackerel, about 175g/6oz each,
   cleaned, gutted/dressed, boned
   and heads removed
juice of ½ lemon
freshly ground black pepper
1 lemon, cut into wedges, to serve

STUFFING
2 tsp sunflower oil
1 small onion, finely chopped
25g/1oz brown rice, cooked
juice and zest of ½ lemon
1 tbsp finely chopped parsley
   leaves
1 small egg, beaten
2.5cm/1in piece of root ginger,
   peeled and finely chopped
salad, to serve

1 Preheat the oven to 160°C/325°F/Gas 3. To make the stuffing, heat the oil in a saucepan over a medium heat until hot. Add the onion and cook for 5 minutes, or until translucent. Transfer to a mixing bowl, add the cooked rice and the remaining stuffing ingredients and mix together.

2 Put the mackerel on a work surface, sprinkle the lemon juice over the top and season with black pepper. Spoon the stuffing into the centre of the fish, then tie the fish to prevent the stuffing falling out while cooking.

3 Put the fish in an ovenproof dish and pour in 3 tablespoons of water. Cover with a lid and bake for 15–20 minutes, or until thoroughly cooked through. Serve hot with lemon and salad.

Pictured right

Poached Halibut with Parsley Sauce

1 small leek, chopped
1 carrot, chopped
2 tbsp finely chopped parsley
   leaves
4 halibut steaks
juice of 1 lemon
new potatoes and green beans,
   to serve

1 Cover the bottom of a large saucepan with the leek and carrot and sprinkle 1 tablespoon of the parsley over the top. Put the steaks on top and pour the lemon juice and 150ml/5fl oz/scant ⅔ cup water over them.

2 Bring to the boil over a medium heat, cover with a lid, and simmer for 10 minutes, or until thoroughly cooked. Transfer the fish to a serving dish and keep warm.

3 Turn the heat up again and bring the liquid and vegetables back to the boil. Simmer for a further 5 minutes, or until the vegetables are soft.

4 Put the vegetables in a blender or food processor and blend until smooth. Return to the saucepan, add the remaining tablespoon of parsley and continue to cook until the liquid reduces to a thick sauce.

5 Serve the fish with the sauce poured over the top, along with new potatoes and green beans.

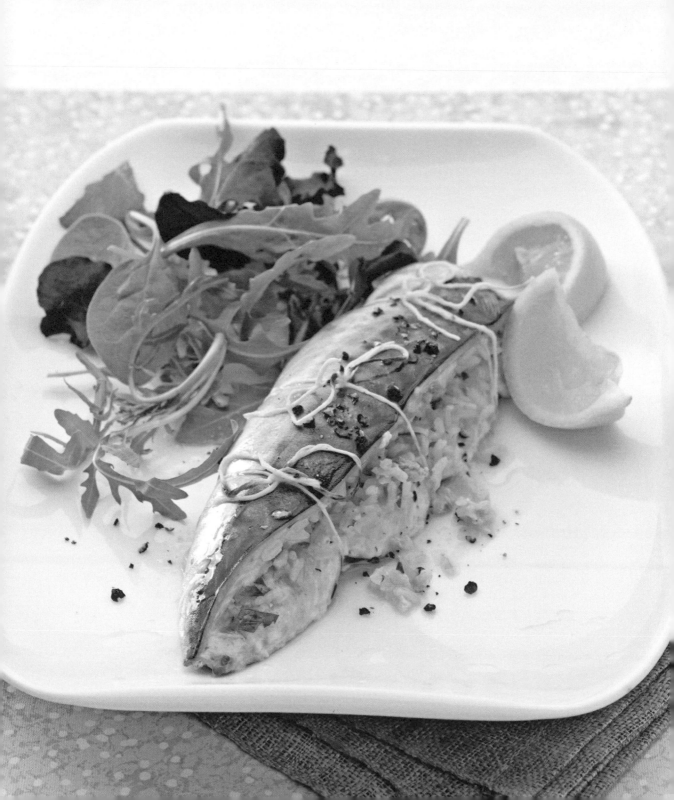

Sweet Soy Sauce Fish with Spinach

2 tsp sesame oil
4 tilapia fish fillets
500ml/17fl oz/2 cups chicken stock
4 tbsp soy sauce
1 tsp honey
16 large handfuls of spinach leaves
4 garlic cloves, finely chopped
2 red chillies, deseeded and
  finely chopped
2 tbsp tamari soy sauce
salad, to serve

1 Heat the oil in a large frying pan over a high heat until hot. Add the fish and sear on each side for 2–3 minutes until just cooked, adding a little stock if necessary.

2 Stir the soy sauce into the honey. Reduce the heat to medium and pour in the soy sauce and honey mixture, and half of the stock. Heat through until the fish is glazed by the sauce.

3 Meanwhile, put the spinach in a wok and add the garlic, chillies, tamari and remaining stock. Stir and cook for 4 minutes, or until the spinach wilts.

4 Divide the spinach into bowls, top with the fish and serve immediately with salad.

Tuna & Fennel Pasta Bake

250g/8oz white pasta shells
1 tbsp sunflower oil
1 fennel bulb, trimmed and finely
  sliced
1 onion, finely sliced
3 eggs
200g/7oz canned tuna, drained
  and flaked
50g/1¾oz mature Cheddar
  cheese, grated
freshly ground black pepper

WHITE SAUCE
600ml/21fl oz/scant 2½ cups
  semi-skimmed/2% milk
50g/1¾oz cornflour/cornstarch

1 Bring a large saucepan of water to the boil over a high heat. Add the pasta and cook over a medium heat for a few minutes less than the package advises (the pasta will finish cooking in the oven). Drain and set aside.

2 Meanwhile, heat the oil in a large frying pan over a medium heat. Add the onion and fennel and cook for 3–5 minutes until soft but not coloured. Set aside.

3 Put the eggs in a small saucepan and cover with cold water. Bring to the boil over a high heat, then reduce the heat to low and simmer for 5 minutes. Drain the water from the pan and then leave it to stand under cold running water for 1 minute. Leave the eggs in the pan of cold water for a further 2 minutes, then peel and set aside to cool before coarsely chopping.

4 Preheat the oven to 200°C/400°F/Gas 6. To make the sauce, heat the milk in a large saucepan over a medium heat until almost boiling, then remove from the heat. Add 1 tablespoon of water to the cornflour/cornstarch in a small bowl and stir to form a smooth paste. Gradually whisk the paste into the milk, stirring continuously for 2–3 minutes until thick. Stir in the pasta, fennel, onion, eggs, tuna and half the cheese and season with pepper.

5 Put the mixture in a shallow ovenproof dish and sprinkle with the remaining cheese. Bake for 30 minutes, or until golden brown on top. Serve hot.

Salmon Steaks with Ginger

4 salmon steaks
juice of 1 lemon
2.5cm/1in piece of root ginger,
  peeled and finely chopped
2 handfuls of dill, chopped
freshly ground black pepper
new potatoes and green beans,
  to serve

1 Preheat the oven to 180°C/350°F/Gas 4. Put each salmon steak on a piece of baking parchment and sprinkle with the lemon juice and ginger. Sprinkle with the dill and season with pepper.

2 Wrap the parchment around the salmon and bake for 20 minutes, or until cooked through.

3 Serve the salmon hot with new potatoes and green beans.

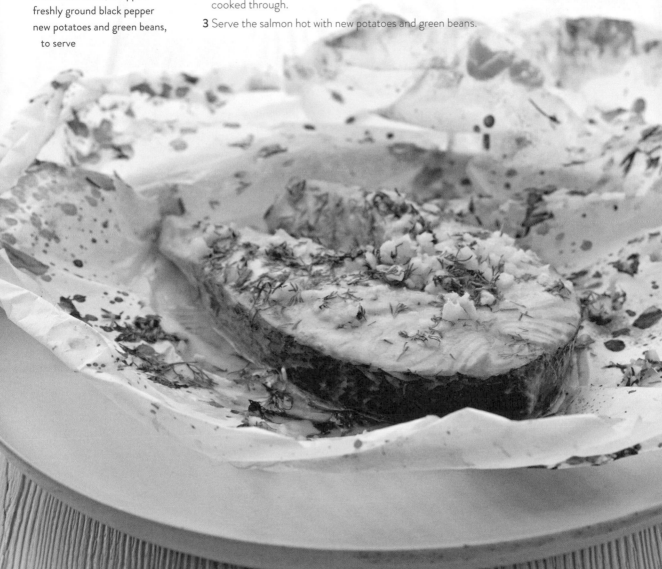

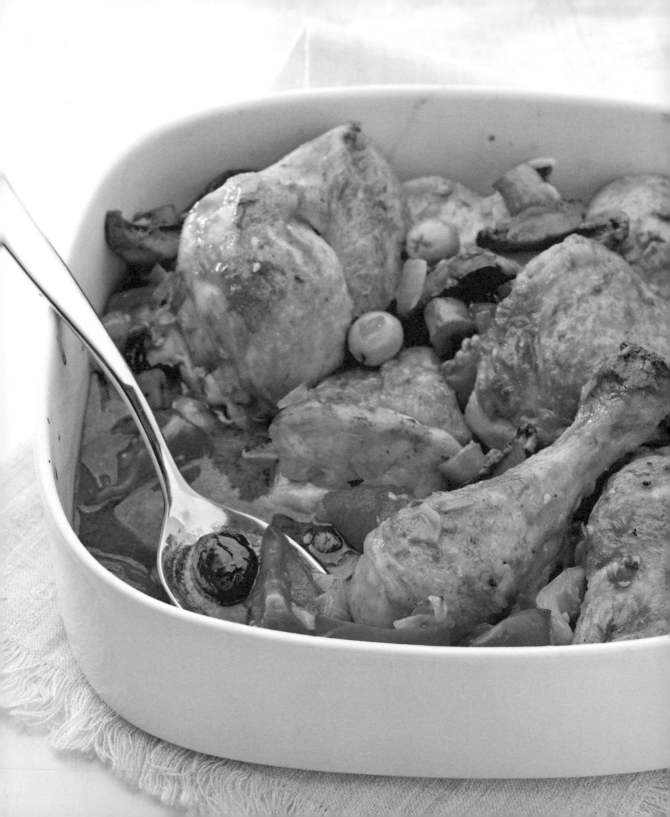

Spanish Chicken

2 tbsp sunflower oil
1 chicken, cut into portions
1 large onion, finely chopped
1 green pepper, deseeded and cut
   into strips
1 red pepper, deseeded and cut
   into strips
225g/8oz mushrooms, sliced
10 pitted green olives
10 pitted black olives
6 tomatoes, chopped
300ml/10½fl oz/scant 1¼ cups
   chicken stock
rice, to serve

1 Heat half the oil in a frying pan over a medium heat until hot and fry the chicken pieces for 5 minutes, or until light brown all over. Remove the chicken from the pan with a slotted spoon, transfer to an ovenproof dish and set aside.

2 Add the onion, peppers, mushrooms, olives and tomatoes to the frying pan. Turn the heat down to low, and fry, stirring occasionally for 5 minutes until soft. Remove the vegetables with a slotted spoon and spoon them over the chicken.

3 Preheat the oven to 180°C/350°F/Gas 4. Heat the stock in a saucepan until boiling. Pour it over the chicken, cover the dish with a lid and bake for 1–1½ hours, until the chicken is cooked through.

4 Remove from the oven and serve hot with rice.

Pictured left

Creamy Chicken Curry

1 tbsp vegetable oil
1 onion, finely chopped
2 garlic cloves, crushed
1cm/½in piece of root ginger,
   peeled and grated
2 tbsp curry powder
1 tbsp white wine vinegar
4 chicken breasts
150ml/5fl oz/scant ⅔ cup
   unsweetened soy milk
150ml/5fl oz/scant ⅔ cup
   coconut cream
1 tbsp sesame seeds
rice, to serve

1 Heat the oil in a flameproof casserole dish over a low heat until hot. Add the onion, garlic and ginger and cook for 8–10 minutes, stirring frequently.

2 Turn up the heat to high, add the curry powder and white wine vinegar and cook for 1 minute until the ingredients have blended.

3 Add the chicken, then pour in the milk and coconut cream and mix well. Bring to the boil, reduce the heat to low, cover with a lid and simmer for 20–30 minutes, until the chicken is cooked through. Sprinkle the sesame seeds over the top and serve hot with rice.

Thai Green Chicken Curry

1 tbsp vegetable oil
500g/1lb 2oz chicken breasts, thinly sliced
140ml/4½fl oz/½ cup coconut cream
250ml/9fl oz/1 cup unsweetened soy milk
1 tbsp Thai fish sauce
225g/8oz tinned sliced bamboo shoots, drained and rinsed
125g/4½oz baby corn cobs
100g/3½oz mangetout/snow peas, trimmed (optional)
100g/3½oz/2 cups basil leaves (optional)
finely sliced green chillies and jasmine rice, to serve

THAI GREEN CURRY PASTE
3 green chillies, deseeded and roughly chopped, plus extra, finely sliced, to serve
1 shallot, roughly chopped
2.5cm/1in piece of root ginger, peeled and roughly chopped
1 garlic clove, crushed
2 handfuls of coriander/cilantro leaves
1 lemongrass stalk, roughly chopped
juice and zest of 1 lime
8 kaffir lime leaves or zest of 1 lime
2 tsp ground coriander/cilantro
½ tsp ground cumin
½ tsp freshly ground black pepper
1 tsp shrimp paste
1 tsp light soy sauce
2 tbsp olive oil

1 To make the curry paste, put all the ingredients in a blender or food processor and blend to a paste.

2 Heat the oil in a frying pan over a medium heat until hot. Add the chicken and cook, stirring continuously, for 5 minutes, or until brown all over.

3 Stir 3 tablespoons of the curry paste into the chicken and then pour in the coconut cream, soy milk and fish sauce and bring to the boil, stirring occasionally. (Store the remaining curry paste in the refrigerator for up to 2 days or in the freezer for up to 3 months.)

4 Reduce the heat to medium, add the bamboo shoots and corn and cook for 20 minutes, or until the corn is just tender and the chicken is cooked through.

5 Remove the pan from the heat and stir in the mangetout/snow peas (if using) and basil. Sprinkle with finely sliced green chillies and serve immediately with rice.

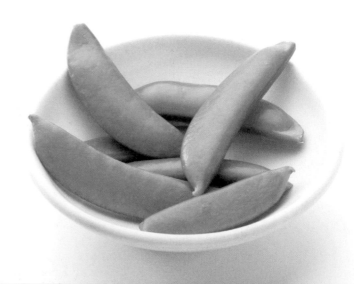

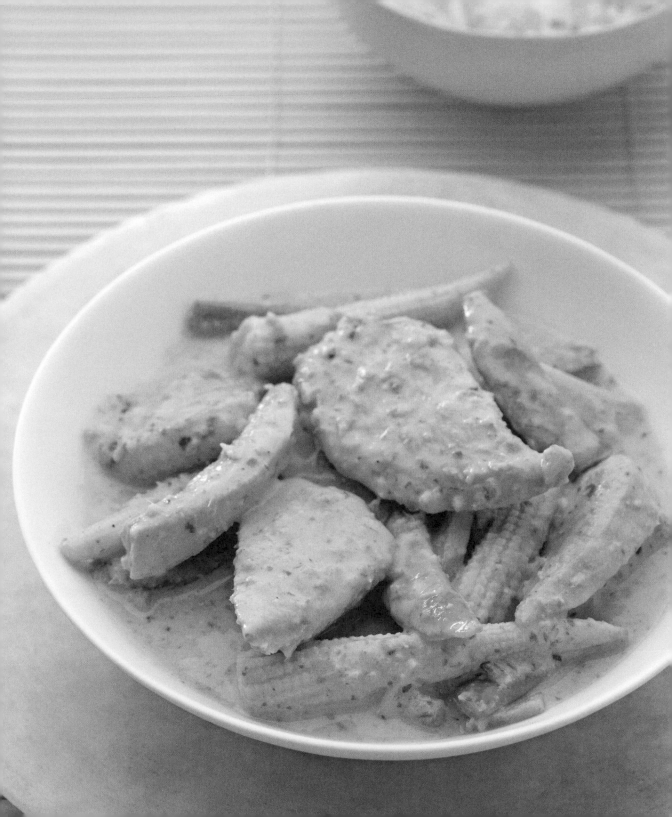

Yogurt Roast Chicken

225ml/7¾fl oz/scant 1 cup
   plain yogurt
2 tsp curry powder
1 large handful of coriander/
   cilantro leaves, finely chopped
5cm/2in piece of root ginger,
   peeled and grated
3 garlic cloves, crushed
4 chicken quarters
baked potatoes and salad, to serve

1 In a small bowl, mix together the yogurt, curry powder, coriander/cilantro, ginger and garlic. Pour the mixture all over the chicken, making sure it is completely coated, then cover and refrigerate for 1–2 hours.
2 Preheat the oven to 180°C/350°F/Gas 4. Put the chicken and yogurt sauce in a roasting pan, spooning the sauce over the chicken so it is covered. Bake with a lid on for 1½ hours, or until the chicken is cooked through.
3 Transfer the chicken to a serving dish and keep warm. Pour the yogurt sauce and the chicken juices into a saucepan and bring to the boil over a high heat and boil until reduced. Pour the sauce over the chicken and serve immediately with baked potatoes and salad.

Beef Stir-Fry with Apricot & Walnut

6 fresh apricots, pitted and cut
   into quarters, or unsulphured
   dried apricots
350g/12oz rump/sirloin steak,
   fat removed
2 tsp cornflour/cornstarch
4 tbsp orange juice
2 tsp groundnut/peanut or
   vegetable oil
4 spring onions/scallions, sliced
   diagonally into 2.5cm/1in pieces
1 tbsp Worcestershire sauce
3 Chinese leaves, roughly chopped
50g/1¾oz/scant ½ cup walnut
   pieces
freshly ground black pepper
noodles or rice, to serve

1 If using dried apricots, soak in a bowl of cold water for 1 hour, then drain and cut into quarters.
2 Wrap the steak in cling film/plastic wrap and freeze for 45 minutes, or until nearly frozen. Remove the meat from the freezer, take off the cling film/plastic wrap and cut across the grain into very thin strips.
3 In a small jug, mix together the cornflour/cornstarch and 1 tablespoon of water until it forms a smooth paste. Pour in 4 more tablespoons of water and the orange juice and mix thoroughly, then set aside.
4 Heat the oil in a wok or frying pan over a high heat until hot. Add the meat and stir-fry for 3 minutes, or until brown. Reduce the heat to medium, add the spring onions/scallions, Worcestershire sauce and Chinese leaves and continue to stir-fry for a further 1 minute, or until the onions are translucent. Add the apricots and the cornflour/cornstarch mixture to the pan. Bring to the boil over a medium to high heat, stirring continuously. After about 30 seconds, the mixture should become thick and glossy.
5 Remove the pan from the heat and stir in the walnuts. Season with pepper and serve immediately with noodles or rice.

Pictured right

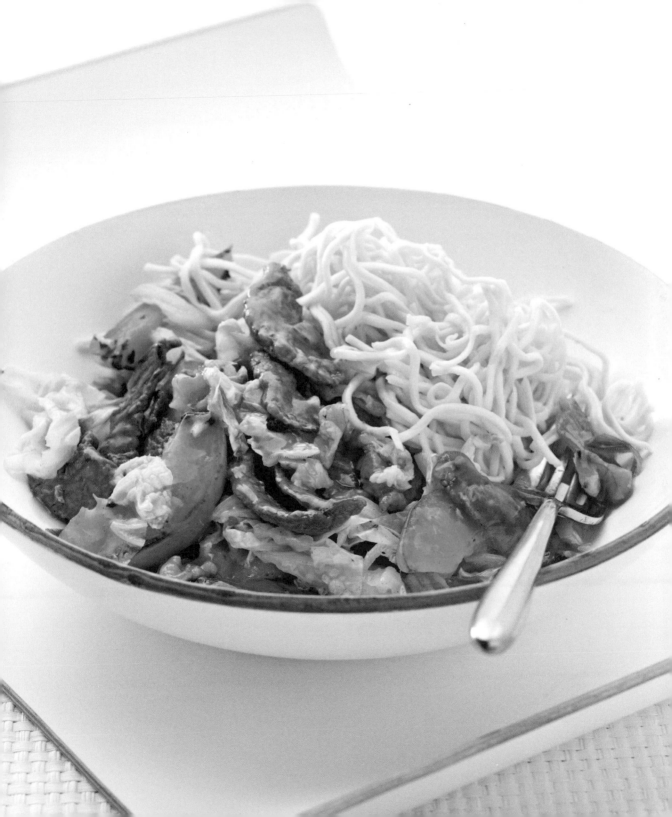

Individual Moussakas

1 aubergine/eggplant, sliced
lengthways into 8 slices
olive oil, for rubbing and greasing
salad, to serve

MEAT SAUCE
1 tbsp olive oil
1 onion, finely chopped
2 garlic cloves, chopped
500g/1lb 2oz minced/ground beef
1 tbsp chopped oregano leaves
½ tsp cinnamon
375ml/13fl oz/1½ cups passata
125ml/4fl oz/½ cup red wine
1 tsp brown sugar
freshly ground black pepper

WHITE SAUCE
60g/2¼oz butter
2 tbsp plain/all-purpose flour
375ml/13fl oz/1½ cups
unsweetened soy milk
1 egg, beaten

1 Preheat the grill/broiler to medium. Spray the aubergine/eggplant slices with oil and grill/broil for 1 minute on each side or until soft and charred. Remove from the oven and set aside.

2 To make the meat sauce, heat the oil in a frying pan over a medium heat until hot. Add the onion and garlic and fry for 3 minutes, or until soft, stirring frequently. Stir in the beef and continue to fry, stirring continuously for 5 minutes, or until brown. Add the oregano, cinnamon, passata and wine. Bring to the boil and then reduce the heat to low and simmer for 20 minutes, or until the sauce is reduced and thickened. Add the sugar and season with pepper.

3 Meanwhile, make the white sauce. Melt the butter in a small saucepan over a medium heat. Add the flour and stir for 1–2 minutes, using a wooden spoon, until the ingredients have blended. Remove the pan from the heat and gradually stir in the soy milk until smooth and creamy. Return to the heat and slowly bring to the boil, or until it begins to bubble, stirring continuously. Simmer slowly for 3 minutes, stirring continuously, or until the sauce thickens. Remove from the heat and add the egg. Whisk thoroughly until the sauce is fully blended.

4 Preheat the oven to 180°C/350°F/Gas 4 and grease 4 x 250ml/9fl oz/ 1 cup baking dishes or ramekins with olive oil. Put 1 slice of aubergine/ eggplant on the bottom of each dish, then pour a quarter of the meat sauce over it. Add another slice of aubergine/eggplant, then add a quarter of the white sauce. Bake for about 15 minutes until golden brown. Serve warm with a salad.

Lamb's Liver with Orange

2 tbsp cornflour/cornstarch
2 tbsp plain/all-purpose flour
350g/12oz lamb's liver, thinly
sliced
2 tbsp sunflower oil
2 onions, thinly sliced
1 green pepper, deseeded and
diced
150g/5oz lean back/Canadian
bacon, sliced
230ml/7¾fl oz/1 cup orange juice
4 oranges, peeled, separated into
segments and cut in half
freshly ground black pepper
selection of vegetables, to serve

1 Put the cornflour/cornstarch and plain/all-purpose flour in a bowl, season with black pepper and mix together thoroughly. Dip each piece of liver into the flour until well coated.

2 Heat the oil in a frying pan over a medium heat until hot. Add the onion and fry for 4–5 minutes, stirring occasionally, until translucent. Add the pepper, bacon and liver and fry for a further 8 minutes, or until the meat is cooked through.

3 Pour in the orange juice and simmer for 5 minutes, or until the ingredients are soft. Add the orange segments and cook for a further 1 minute until heated through. Serve with vegetables.

Lamb & Aubergine Bake

4 aubergines/eggplants, cut in
half lengthways
50g/1¾oz/¼ cup brown rice
4 tsp sunflower oil
2 small onions, finely chopped
2 garlic cloves, finely chopped
1 tbsp canned sweetcorn/corn
kernels, drained and rinsed
200g/7oz minced/ground lamb
1 tbsp tomato purée/paste
freshly ground black pepper
brown rice and salad, to serve

1 Preheat the oven to 190°C/375°F/Gas 5. Scoop out the aubergine/eggplant flesh using a spoon, leaving enough around the edges so the shells hold their shape. Set the shells aside and chop the flesh.

2 Put the rice in a saucepan, cover with water, bring to the boil, then reduce the heat and simmer for 25 minutes until tender. Drain and set aside.

3 Heat the oil in a frying pan over a moderate heat until hot. Add the onion and garlic and fry for 4–5 minutes, stirring occasionally, until the onions are translucent. Add the chopped aubergine/eggplant and continue to fry for a further 2 minutes, stirring frequently.

4 Add the rice, corn, lamb and tomato purée/paste to the pan, season with pepper and, continuing to stir, fry for 3 minutes or until the meat is brown.

5 Spoon the mixture into the aubergine/eggplant halves. Put in a covered ovenproof dish and bake for 20–25 minutes, or until the aubergines/eggplants are cooked through. Serve hot with brown rice and salad.

Pork with Orange & Herb Sauce

2 tsp sunflower oil
1 small onion, finely chopped
2 boneless pork loin steaks, diced
2 tsp chopped tarragon leaves
2 tsp chopped parsley leaves, plus
  extra to serve
175ml/6fl oz/¾ cup orange juice
2 tsp cornflour/cornstarch
1 orange, peeled, separated into
  segments and chopped
freshly ground black pepper
selection of vegetables, to serve

1 Heat the oil in a frying pan over a medium heat until hot. Add the onion and fry for 3 minutes, or until translucent, stirring occasionally. Add the pork and fry for 10 minutes, or until cooked through, stirring occasionally.

2 Add the tarragon, parsley and orange juice and season with pepper. Turn the heat to high and bring to the boil, then reduce the heat to medium until gently bubbling, and simmer for 2–3 minutes.

3 In a small bowl, mix the cornflour/cornstarch with 1 tablespoon water and stir until it forms a smooth paste. Add to the sauce and bring to the boil, stirring continuously. Reduce the heat, add the orange segments and cook for 1–2 minutes until the orange is soft. Sprinkle with extra parsley and serve with vegetables.

Pictured right

Noodles in Spicy Sesame Sauce

450g/1lb rice noodles
150ml/5fl oz/scant ⅔ cup sesame
  oil
3 garlic cloves, finely chopped
5cm/2in piece of root ginger,
  peeled and finely grated
5 spring onions/scallions,
  finely chopped
1 tsp chilli powder/cayenne pepper
150ml/5fl oz/scant ⅔ cup tahini
2 tbsp tamari soy sauce
3 tbsp rice vinegar
1 tbsp tomato purée/paste
1 large tomato, diced
freshly ground black pepper

1 Bring a large saucepan of water to the boil. Drop in the noodles, turn off the heat and leave to stand for 5 minutes, stirring occasionally.

2 Heat the oil in a saucepan over a medium heat until hot and fry the garlic and ginger for 3 minutes, or until soft, stirring continuously. Add the spring onions/scallions and fry for a further 3 minutes, or until cooked through, then add the chilli powder/cayenne, season with pepper and fry for a further 1 minute. Stir continuously.

3 Pour 150ml/5fl oz/scant ⅔ cup cold water into a bowl and add the tahini, tamari, rice vinegar and tomato purée/paste. Mix together thoroughly until the ingredients have blended, then pour into the saucepan. Turn the heat to high and bring to the boil, then reduce the heat to medium and simmer for 5 minutes.

4 Serve the noodles with the sauce and the tomato pieces sprinkled over the top.

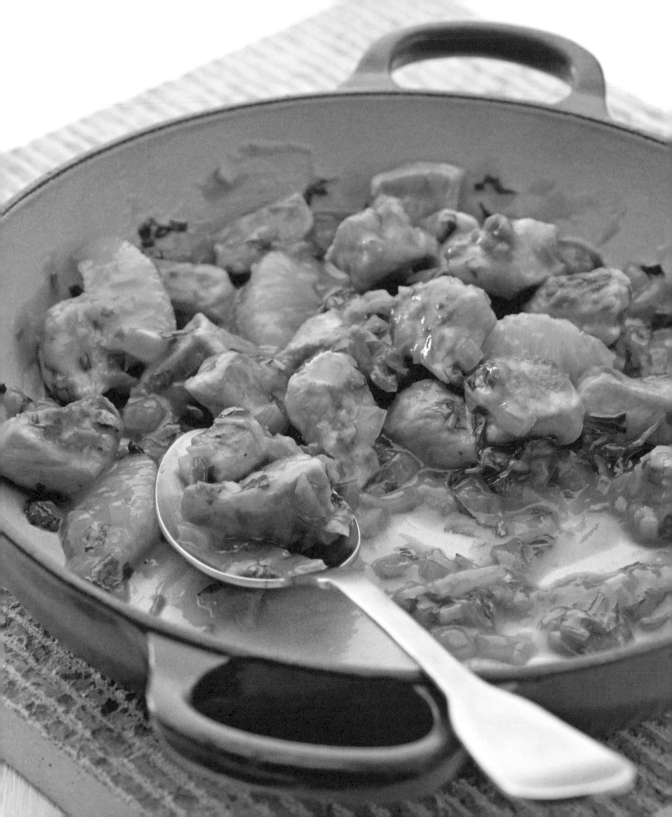

Indonesian Tofu Kebabs with Satay Sauce

550g/1lb 4oz firm tofu, cut into
  2.5cm/1in cubes
4 tbsp tamari soy sauce
2 tbsp clear honey
2 tbsp soy oil
2 garlic cloves, crushed
8 shallots, halved
2 red peppers, deseeded and cut
  into chunks
rice, to serve

SATAY SAUCE
2 tbsp soy oil
2 shallots, finely chopped
1–2 green chillies, deseeded and
  finely chopped
½ tsp ground cumin
½ tsp cayenne pepper
50g/1¾oz creamed coconut
125g/4½oz/½ cup crunchy peanut
  butter
2 tbsp tamari soy sauce

1 Put the tofu in a dish and pour 2 tablespoons of the tamari over it. Cover and leave to marinate for 30 minutes.

2 Preheat the grill/broiler to medium. In a bowl, mix together the remaining tamari, honey, oil and garlic and set aside. Thread the tofu cubes, shallot halves and red pepper chunks onto skewers, then dip each skewer into the tamari and honey mixture, coating them evenly.

3 Heat the oil for the satay sauce in a frying pan over a medium heat until hot. Add the shallots, chillies, cumin and cayenne pepper and fry for 3 minutes, or until soft, stirring occasionally.

4 Put the kebabs on a grill/broiler pan and grill for about 10 minutes, turning frequently, until brown.

5 In a bowl, dissolve the creamed coconut in 150ml/5fl oz/scant ⅔ cup boiling water. Add to the frying pan along with the peanut butter and tamari. Stir well and cook for 3 minutes, or until hot. Drizzle the sauce over the kebabs and serve with rice.

Lasagne

100g/3½oz soy mince/ground "meat" TVP
1 tbsp soy oil
1 onion, finely chopped
2 garlic cloves, crushed
400g/14oz canned chopped tomatoes
250ml/9fl oz/1 cup passata
75g/2½oz mushrooms, sliced
2 tbsp red wine
1 small handful of oregano leaves, chopped
4 bay leaves
1 small handful of basil leaves, chopped
1 tsp paprika
1 tsp sugar
soy margarine, for greasing
12 pre-cooked lasagne sheets
freshly ground black pepper
salad, to serve

CHEESE SAUCE
50g/1¾oz soy margarine
1 tbsp cornflour/cornstarch
550ml/19fl oz/scant 2¼ cups unsweetened soy milk
75g/2¾oz Cheddar cheese, grated
freshly ground black pepper

1 Put the soy mince/TVP in a bowl and pour 550ml/19fl oz/scant 2¼ cups of water over the top. Leave to stand for 15 minutes, or until the water has been absorbed.

2 Heat the oil in a large saucepan over a medium heat until hot. Add the onion and garlic and fry for 4–5 minutes, stirring occasionally, until soft. Stir in the soy mince/TVP, tomatoes, passata, mushrooms, red wine, herbs, paprika and sugar. Season with pepper and simmer gently for 15 minutes, or until cooked through. Remove the bay leaves and set the sauce to one side.

3 Meanwhile, make the cheese sauce. Melt the margarine in a saucepan over a medium heat, stir in the cornflour/cornstarch and cook for 1 minute. Remove the pan from the heat and gradually stir in the milk until smooth and creamy. Return to the heat and slowly bring to the boil, stirring continuously, until thoroughly blended. Reduce the heat to low and simmer slowly for about 3 minutes, stirring all the time, until the sauce is thick and smooth. Stir in two-thirds of the cheese and season with pepper.

4 Preheat the oven to 200°C/400°F/Gas 6 and grease a 30 x 26cm/12 x 10in ovenproof dish with soy margarine. Spread half of the soy mince/TVP sauce over the bottom of the dish, then cover with a layer of 4 lasagne sheets and drizzle half of the cheese sauce over the top. Layer again and use the remaining lasagne sheets to cover the top. Sprinkle the remaining Cheddar cheese over the lasagne and bake for about 30 minutes until golden. Serve hot with salad.

Red Lentil & Coconut Cream

225g/8oz/scant 1 cup split red
   lentils
4 large carrots, chopped
1 onion, finely chopped
1 garlic clove, crushed
1 tsp paprika
½ tsp ground ginger
1 bay leaf
15g/½oz creamed coconut, grated
2 tbsp lemon juice
freshly ground black pepper
rice and vegetables, to serve

1 Wash the lentils and put in a large saucepan. Add the carrots, onion, garlic, paprika, ginger, bay leaf and 550ml/19fl oz/scant 2¼ cups cold water.

2 Bring to the boil over a medium heat, then, using a metal spoon, skim the surface to remove any scum. Reduce the heat to low, cover with a lid and simmer for 25–30 minutes until most of the water has been absorbed.

3 Remove the bay leaf and mash the mixture into a smooth paste with a hand masher. Stir in the creamed coconut and lemon juice and season with pepper. Serve hot with rice and vegetables.

Tofu "Meatballs"

½ tsp olive oil, for greasing
1 onion, roughly chopped
4 large handfuls of parsley,
   roughly chopped
275g/9¾oz tofu
50g/1¾oz/scant ⅔ cup
   breadcrumbs
1 egg
1 handful of basil leaves
1 handful of oregano leaves
1 tsp ground nutmeg
1 garlic clove
50g/1¾oz Parmesan cheese,
   grated
250ml/9fl oz/1 cup passata
2 tbsp soy flour
freshly ground black pepper
rice and vegetables, to serve

1 Preheat the oven to 180°C/350°F/Gas 4 and grease a baking sheet with olive oil. Put the onion and parsley in a blender or food processor and blend until smooth. Add the tofu, breadcrumbs, egg, herbs, nutmeg, garlic, cheese and 3 tablespoons of the passata. Blend until all the ingredients are combined into a smooth mixture.

2 Shape the tofu mixture into balls using a dessertspoon, then dip each ball into the flour to coat. Put the tofu balls on the baking sheet and bake for 35 minutes, or until golden and crisp on the outside.

3 Remove from the oven and transfer to a large saucepan. Add the remaining passata and place the pan over a medium heat. Cover with a lid and simmer for 10 minutes, or until the sauce is hot. Serve hot with rice and vegetables.

Tofu & Vegetable Rice

225g/8oz/heaped 1 cup long-grain brown rice
50g/1¾oz green beans
100g/3½oz carrots, cut into matchsticks
100g/3½oz courgettes/zucchini, cut into matchsticks
100g/3½oz broccoli florets
1 tbsp soy oil
225g/8oz firm tofu, cut into 2.5cm/1in cubes
1 onion, finely chopped
1 garlic clove, finely chopped
1 red pepper, deseeded and cut into strips
1 green pepper, deseeded and cut into strips
1 small orange, peeled and broken into segments
1 tbsp flaked/sliced almonds
1 tbsp finely chopped parsley leaves

1 Put the rice in a saucepan and cover with water. Bring to the boil and then turn down the heat to low and simmer, covered, for 25 minutes, or until tender. Drain and set aside, keeping the lid on to contain the heat.

2 While the rice is cooking, put the beans, carrots, courgettes and broccoli in a steamer and cook for 5 minutes, or until they are cooked through but still firm.

3 Heat the oil in a large frying pan over a medium heat until hot. Add the tofu, onion, garlic and peppers and fry for 3 minutes, or until the onions are translucent, stirring frequently.

4 Stir in the steamed vegetables together with the orange, almonds, parsley and rice. Heat through while stirring continuously. Season with pepper and serve.

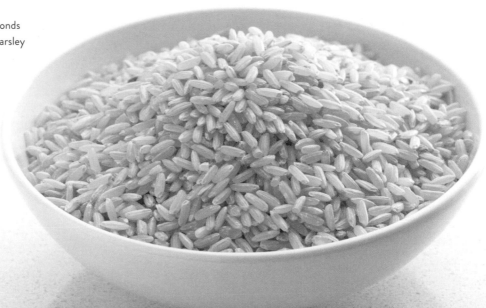

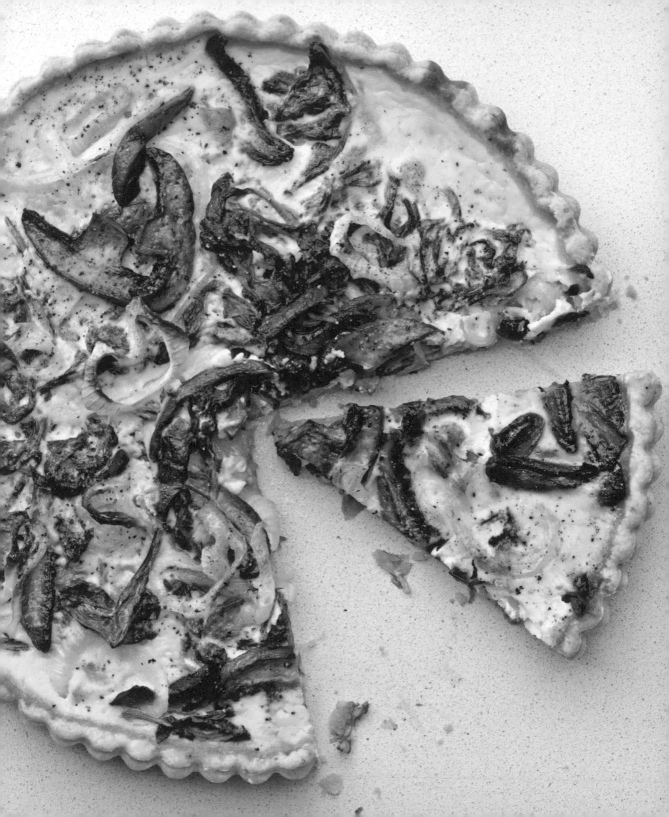

Spanish Omelette Bake

8 potatoes, diced
8 carrots, diced
115g/4oz broccoli florets
2 leeks, sliced
4 eggs, beaten
200ml/7 fl oz/¾ cup plus 1 tbsp
  unsweetened soy milk
1 tsp finely chopped chives
1 garlic clove, crushed
2 large tomatoes, sliced
55g/2oz vegetarian cheese, grated
½ tsp olive oil, for greasing
freshly ground black pepper
salad, to serve

1 Put the potatoes and carrots in a large saucepan and cover with cold water. Bring to the boil over a high heat, reduce the heat to medium and simmer for 5 minutes, or until they start to cook. Add the broccoli and leeks and simmer for a further 5 minutes, or until they are just cooked. Alternatively, put the broccoli and leeks in a steamer over the saucepan and cook for 5 minutes, or until cooked through but firm. Drain the vegetables.

2 Preheat the oven to 180°C/350°F/Gas 4 and grease a 20cm/8in ovenproof dish with the olive oil. Whisk the egg and milk together in a jug, then mix in the chives and garlic and season with pepper. Put the vegetables into the dish and pour the egg mixture over, then cover with a layer of tomatoes and sprinkle them with the cheese. Bake for 35–40 minutes, or until golden brown and set. Serve hot with salad.

Mushroom & Spinach Quiche

1 tbsp vegetable oil, plus extra for
  greasing
plain/all-purpose flour, for dusting
225g/8oz frozen shortcrust/
  piecrust pastry dough, thawed
100g/3½oz mushrooms, sliced
1 onion, sliced
3 eggs, beaten
150ml/5fl oz/scant ⅔ cup milk
170ml/5½fl oz/scant ⅔ cup natural
  yogurt
225g/8oz frozen spinach, thawed
  and drained
freshly ground black pepper
salad, to serve

1 Preheat the oven to 200°C/400°F/Gas 6 and grease a 24cm/9½in loose-bottomed tart tin with oil. Dust the work surface with flour and roll out the dough into a circle about 30cm/12in in diameter. Using the dusted rolling pin, pick up the dough and gently put it in the tart tin. Press down carefully to remove any air pockets. Line the case with baking parchment and cover with baking beans/pie weights. Bake blind for 10–15 minutes, or until firm to the touch. Remove from the oven, set aside and reduce the oven temperature to 190°C/375°F/Gas 5.

2 Heat the oil in a frying pan over a medium heat until hot. Add the mushrooms and onion and fry for 2–3 minutes until translucent, stirring frequently.

3 In a large bowl, whisk together the eggs and milk, then stir in the yogurt, spinach, mushrooms and onion. Season with pepper.

4 Ladle the mixture into the pastry case/pie-shell and bake for 30 minutes, or until the top looks set. Serve hot with salad.

Pictured left

Spinach & Cheese Soufflé

olive oil, for greasing
50g/1¾oz sunflower margarine
450g/1lb spinach leaves, rinsed
   thoroughly and chopped, or
   225g/8oz frozen spinach,
   thawed
1 garlic clove, finely chopped
3 tbsp brown rice flour
200ml/7fl oz/¾ cup plus 1 tbsp
   semi-skimmed/2% milk
3 eggs, separated, plus 1 egg white
100g/3½oz Gruyère or Cheddar
   cheese, grated
a pinch of ground nutmeg
freshly ground black pepper
salad, to serve

1 Preheat the oven to 190°C/375°F/Gas 5 and grease 4 medium-size ramekins with olive oil. Melt the margarine in a saucepan over a medium heat, add the spinach and cook for 2 minutes, or until it wilts, turning frequently. Add the garlic and stir for a further 1 minute. Add the rice flour and cook gently for 1 minute, stirring continuously.

2 Remove the pan from the heat and gradually stir in the milk until smooth and creamy. Return the pan to the heat and slowly bring to the boil, stirring continuously, until the ingredients are well blended. Reduce the heat to low and simmer for 3 minutes, or until the sauce is thick and smooth, stirring continuously. Leave to cool slightly for 5 minutes.

3 Using a hand whisk/mixer, beat in the 3 egg yolks, one at a time, then add three-quarters of the cheese. Add the nutmeg, season with pepper and stir thoroughly.

4 In a clean bowl, whisk the 4 egg whites until stiff peaks form. Using a metal spoon, gently fold them into the cheese mixture. Spoon into the ramekins and sprinkle with the remaining cheese.

5 Put the ramekins on a baking sheet and bake for 30 minutes, or until well risen and just set. Serve immediately with salad.

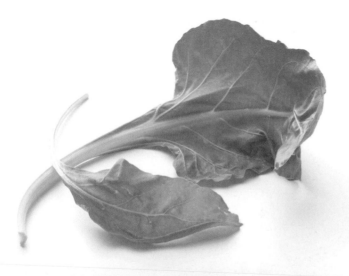

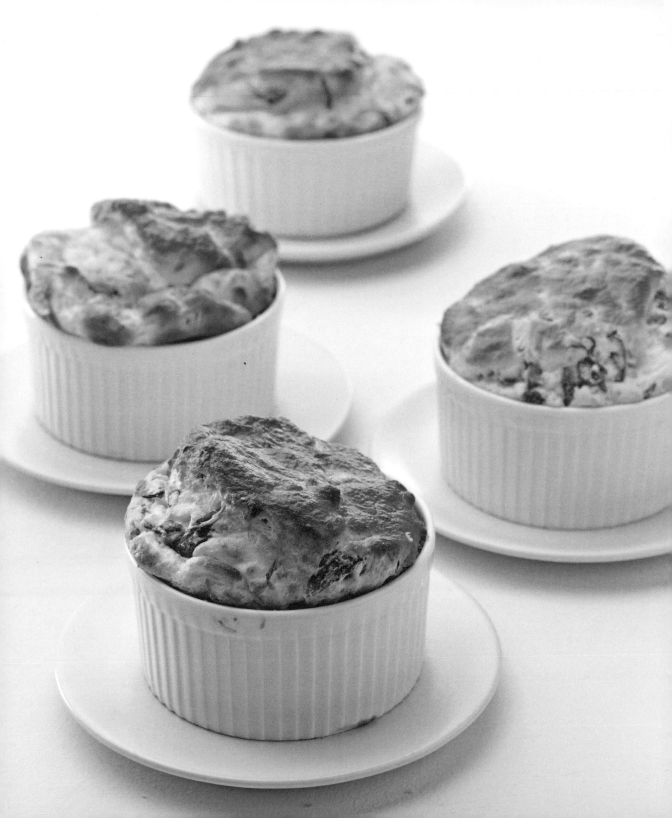

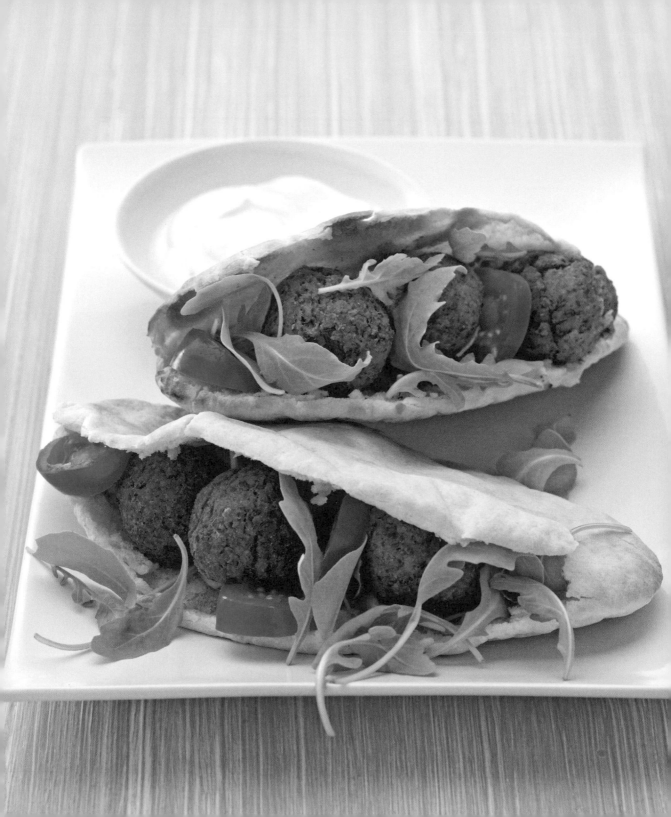

Falafel with Sesame Yogurt Dressing

FALAFEL

400g/14oz canned chickpeas, drained and rinsed

6 spring onions/scallions, finely chopped

30g/1oz/scant ½ cup white breadcrumbs

1 egg, beaten

juice and zest of 1 lemon

1 garlic clove, crushed

2 tbsp finely chopped coriander/cilantro leaves

2 tbsp finely chopped parsley leaves

1 tbsp tahini

1 tsp ground coriander

1 tsp ground cumin

½ tsp cinnamon

a pinch of cayenne pepper

1l/36fl oz/4 cups sunflower oil for deep frying

freshly ground black pepper

pitta bread and salad, to serve

SESAME YOGURT DRESSING

4 tbsp plain yogurt

2 tbsp olive oil

1 tbsp lemon juice

1 tbsp tahini

freshly ground black pepper

1 Put all the ingredients for the falafels in a blender or food processor and blend to a smooth paste. Put the mixture in a bowl, cover with cling film/plastic wrap and leave to stand for at least 30 minutes until set.

2 To make the sesame sauce, put all the ingredients into a bowl and whisk together until smooth. Cover the bowl and chill in the refrigerator.

3 Shape the falafel mixture into balls using a dessertspoon.

4 In a wok, heat the sunflower oil to 190°C/375°F. (To make sure the oil is hot enough, add a little bit of the falafel mixture to it and, if it rises to the surface and is sizzling, the oil is ready.) Working in batches, slip 6 falafels into the wok and cook for 3 minutes, or until golden brown.

5 Lift the falafels out of the oil, using a slotted spoon, and drain on paper towels. Serve warm with salad and pitta bread, and the sesame yogurt dressing on the side.

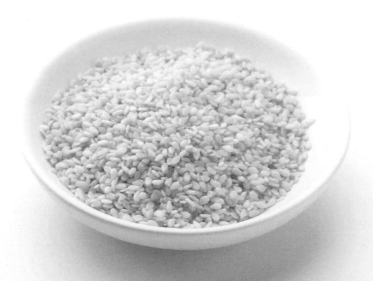

DESSERTS, CAKES, BREADS & SNACKS

Strawberry Soufflé Pancakes

250ml/9floz/1 cup soy milk
2 eggs, separated
zest of 1 lemon
150g/5½oz/scant 1¼ cups
   self-raising/self-rising flour
1 tbsp caster/superfine sugar
1 tsp vanilla extract
500g/1lb 2oz strawberries, hulled
   and halved
3 tbsp clear honey
1 tbsp balsamic vinegar
20g/¾oz butter
icing/confectioners' sugar, to dust

1 To make the batter, whisk together the soy milk, egg yolks, lemon zest, flour, sugar and vanilla extract in a large mixing bowl until smooth. In another clean bowl, whisk the egg whites until stiff peaks form, then use a large metal spoon to gently fold the egg whites into the batter.

2 Put the strawberries in a bowl and pour in the honey and balsamic vinegar. Mix gently with a spoon to coat the fruit.

3 For each pancake, heat a little of the butter in a frying pan over a medium heat until it melts. Pour 2 tablespoons of the batter into the pan and tilt the pan so that the bottom is covered with the mixture. Cook for 2 minutes until the underside of the pancake is golden, then flip over with a spatula and cook for a further 2 minutes until golden and puffed.

4 Remove from the pan and keep warm. Repeat with the remaining batter. Dust with icing/confectioners' sugar and serve warm with the strawberries.

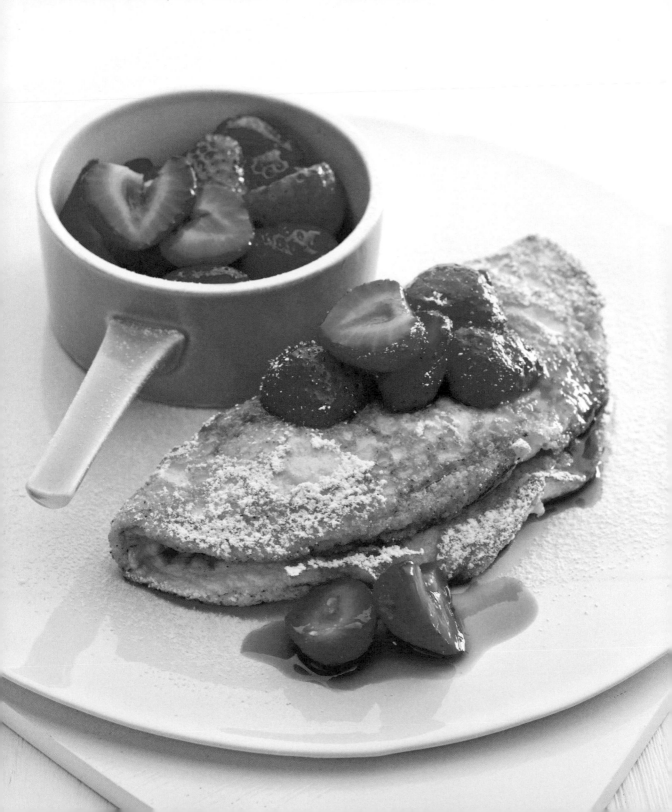

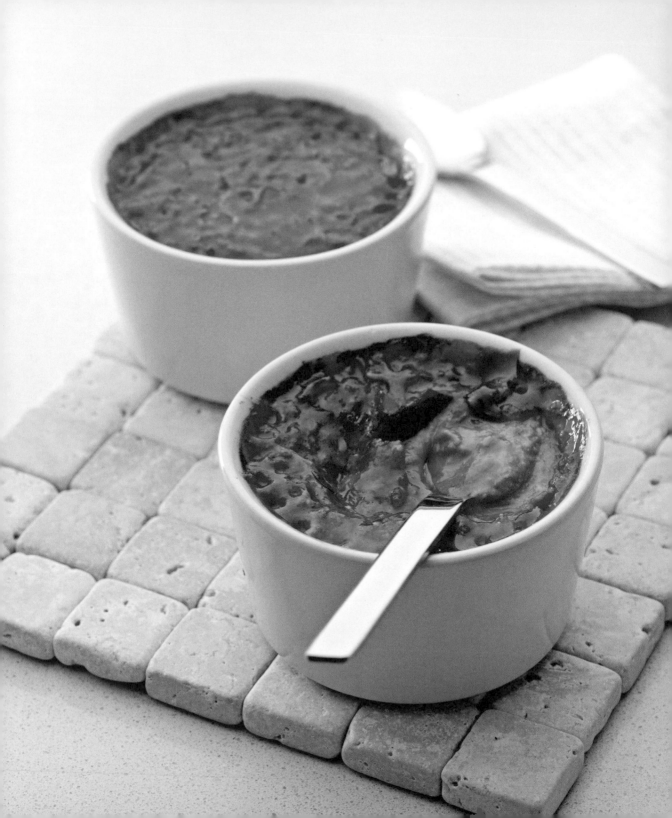

Raspberry & Tofu Brûlée

sunflower oil, to grease
200g/7oz/scant 1⅔ cups
 raspberries
250g/9oz silken tofu
2 tbsp clear honey
3 tbsp golden caster/superfine
 sugar

1 Preheat the grill/broiler to high and grease 4 medium-size ramekin dishes with sunflower oil.
2 Put the raspberries, tofu and honey in a blender or food processor and blend until smooth.
3 Spoon into the ramekins and sprinkle the sugar over the top. Grill/broil for 2–3 minutes or until a golden crust forms. Or use a blow torch to caramelize the sugar so it forms a hard, golden layer. Serve immediately.

Pictured left

Apple & Tofu Cheesecake

SEED PASTRY
soy margarine, for greasing
50g/2oz/scant ⅓ cup chopped
 dried figs
25g/1oz/scant ¼ cup sunflower
 seeds
25g/1oz/¼ cup pumpkin seeds
25g/1oz/¼ cup toasted sesame
 seeds
25g/1oz/scant ¼ cup ground
 hazelnuts
½ tsp mixed/apple pie spice

FILLING
450g/1lb apples, peeled, cored
 and chopped
200g/7oz tofu
1 egg white
2 tbsp lemon juice
1 tsp vanilla extract
1 tsp cinnamon
25g/1oz/¼ cup ground almonds
25g/1oz/¼ cup brown rice flakes

1 Preheat the oven to 180°C/350°F/Gas 4 and grease a 23cm/9in loose-bottom baking pan with margarine The pan should be at least 8cm/3¼in deep. Put the figs and 1 tablespoon boiling water in a bowl. Leave to stand for 10 minutes, or until soft. Transfer to a blender or food processor and blend until smooth.
2 Put the seeds in a mini food processor and process until they form a powder. Transfer to a bowl, add the hazelnuts and mixed spice and mix together. Add the figs and mix in enough cold water to make a dough.
3 Line the base of the baking tin with the dough, using your hands to flatten it. Bake for about 10 minutes until golden. Remove from the oven and set aside.
4 To make the filling, put the apples and tofu in a blender or food processor and pour in 100ml/3½fl oz/scant ½ cup water. Blend to a thick paste and transfer to a large mixing bowl.
5 In another bowl, whisk the egg white until stiff peaks form. Using a large metal spoon, gently fold the egg into the apple mixture. Add the lemon juice, vanilla extract, cinnamon and ground almonds and mix gently. Spoon the mixture onto the pastry case/pie-shell and sprinkle the brown rice flakes over the top.
6 Bake for 30 minutes, or until set.
7 Leave to cool for 5 minutes and then ease out of the pan. Cool completely at room temperature, then chill in the refrigerator. Serve chilled.

Crème Caramel

sunflower oil, for greasing
50g/2oz/¼ cup golden caster/
 superfine sugar, plus 2 tbsp
3 large eggs, beaten
240ml/8fl oz/scant 1 cup
 soy milk
½ tsp vanilla extract
soy cream, to serve

1 Put the sugar in a small saucepan and add 2 tablespoons water. Heat gently over a low heat until the sugar has dissolved. Turn up the heat to medium-high, bring to the boil without stirring and cook for 3 minutes, or until syrupy and a deep golden colour. Remove from the heat and stir in 2 teaspoons boiling water.
2 Preheat the oven to 160°C/325°F/Gas 3 and grease a 600ml/21fl oz/scant 2½ cup ovenproof dish with oil. Pour the sugar syrup into the dish and tilt the dish so the bottom is completely covered.
3 In a bowl, beat the eggs with the soy milk, then add the sugar and vanilla extract and beat again thoroughly. Using a sieve/fine-mesh strainer, strain the mixture into the ovenproof dish and put the dish in a roasting pan. Pour in enough water to come half way up the sides of the ovenproof dish.
4 Bake for 50 minutes, or until set. Remove the dish from the oven and leave to cool for 30 minutes. Turn out onto a serving dish and chill in the refrigerator for 1 hour before serving.

Banana & Rice Pudding

2 bananas, mashed
200g/7oz/scant 1 cup short-grain
 rice
750ml/26fl oz/3 cups soy milk
1 tsp vanilla extract
zest of 1 lemon
1 tsp ground nutmeg
sugar-free jam, to serve

1 Preheat the oven to 180°C/350°F/Gas 4. In a bowl, mix together the bananas, rice, soy milk and vanilla extract until thoroughly combined. Transfer to a 1.75l/60fl oz/scant 7 cup ovenproof dish. Using a fine sieve/strainer, sprinkle the nutmeg over the top.
2 Bake for 1½–2 hours until firm. Serve hot with jam.

Prune & Tofu Dessert

100g/4oz/½ cup pitted prunes
225g/8oz silken tofu
2 tbsp maple syrup
blueberries or strawberries,
  to serve

1 Put the prunes in a bowl and cover with water. Leave to soak for at least 12 hours, or overnight. Drain, put in a saucepan and cover with water. Bring to the boil over a medium heat and simmer for 10–15 minutes until very tender. Drain again, reserving the liquid.

2 Put the prunes in a blender or food processor and add the tofu and maple syrup. While the motor is running, gradually add the cooking juice until a thick, soft purée forms.

3 Transfer to a bowl and chill in the refrigerator for 15 minutes. Serve sprinkled with blueberries or strawberries.

Tofu Strawberry Dessert

15 strawberries, hulled and cut
  vertically into halves
2 tbsp port wine
225g/8oz silken tofu
3 tbsp clear honey
2 tsp vanilla extract
50g/2oz/heaped ½ cup flaked/
  sliced almonds

1 Put the strawberries and port in a bowl and gently mix. Leave to stand for 1 hour, then drain and set aside.

2 Put the tofu in a bowl and mash well with a fork. Add the honey and vanilla extract and mix together.

3 Serve the tofu with the strawberries on top and sprinkled with almonds.

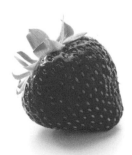
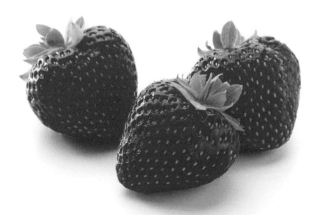

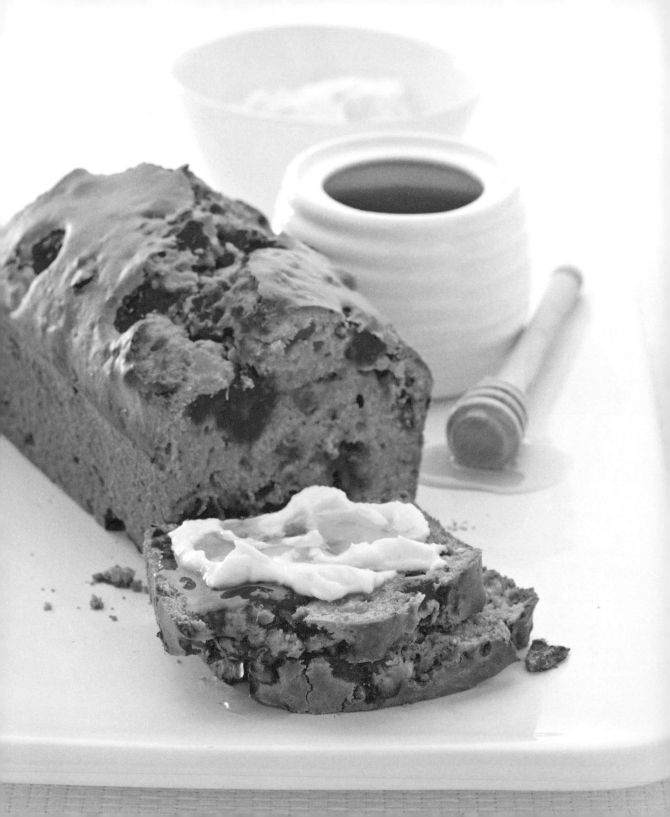

Ginger Fruit Salad

juice of 2 oranges
2 pieces of jarred preserved stem
  ginger, finely chopped, plus 3
  tbsp of the syrup
1 tbsp soft light brown sugar
2 oranges, peeled and pith
  removed
1kg/2lb 4oz honeydew melon
3 apples, peeled, cored and
  chopped
mint leaves, to serve

1 Put the orange juice, stem ginger syrup and sugar in a saucepan. Heat gently over a low heat for 3–4 minutes until the sugar has dissolved. Turn up the heat to medium-high, bring to the boil and cook for 5 minutes, or until syrupy. Remove from the heat and leave to cool for 10 minutes.

2 Slice the oranges into thick rings, then cut the rings into quarters and remove any pips. Cut the melon in half, remove the seeds and scoop out the flesh.

3 Put all the fruit in a serving bowl and pour the ginger syrup over it. Stir well, cover with cling film/plastic wrap and chill in the refrigerator for 1–2 hours. Sprinkle the mint over the top and serve.

Banana & Raspberry Bread

sunflower oil, for greasing
100g/3½oz ripe bananas, mashed
125ml/4floz/½ cup vegetable oil
2 eggs, beaten
90g/3¼oz/ ½ cup soft light brown
  sugar
125ml/4floz/½ cup soy milk
225g/8oz/1¾ cups self-raising/
  self-rising flour
75g/2½oz/scant ⅔ cup plain/
  all-purpose flour
1 tsp ground cinnamon
60g/2¼oz roasted hazelnuts,
  roughly chopped
60g/2¼oz/½ cup dried banana,
  chopped
120g/4¼oz/1 cup raspberries
soy cream cheese and clear honey,
  to serve

1 Preheat the oven to 180°C/350°F/Gas 4 and lightly grease a 22 x 11cm/ 8½ x 4¼in loaf pan with sunflower oil. Beat together the bananas, vegetable oil, eggs, sugar and soy milk in a large mixing bowl.

2 Sift the flours into the mixture and add the cinnamon. Fold together, then add the hazelnuts, dried banana and raspberries and gently fold together.

3 Spoon the mixture into the loaf pan and bake for 1 hour, or until golden and a skewer inserted into the middle comes out clean. Leave the loaf to cool for 5 minutes, then turn out onto a wire rack and leave to cool completely. Serve spread with cream cheese and honey.

Pictured left

Ginger Cake

sunflower oil, for greasing
100g/3½oz sunflower margarine
75g/2½oz/heaped ⅓ cup dark
   muscovado sugar
125ml/4fl oz/½ cup golden syrup
125ml/4fl oz/½ cup treacle
2 tsp ground ginger
½ tsp mixed spice
50g/1¾oz/⅓ cup maize meal
100g/3½oz/heaped ½ cup potato
   flour
100g/3½oz/heaped ½ cup rice
   flour
½ tsp baking powder
2 eggs, beaten
125ml/4fl oz/½ cup milk

1 Preheat the oven to 160°/325°F/Gas 3 and grease a 20cm/8in loose-bottomed cake pan with oil.
2 Melt the margarine and sugar in a saucepan over a medium heat and gradually pour in the golden syrup and treacle and stir in the spices.
3 Sift the maize meal, flours and baking powder into a large mixing bowl and mix together. Make a well in the centre and pour in the syrup mixture. Using a wooden spoon, beat until smooth. In a bowl, beat the eggs and milk, then pour them into the cake mixture, a little at a time, beating continuously to keep the mixture smooth.
4 Pour the mixture into the cake pan and bake for 1 hour, or until cooked through and a skewer inserted into the middle of the cake comes out clean. Leave to cool for 5 minutes, then turn out onto a wire rack and leave to cool completely before serving.

Pictured right

Pineapple Cake

sunflower oil, for greasing
100g/3½oz/heaped ⅓ cup pitted
   and finely chopped prunes
4 tbsp dried figs
300g/10½oz pineapple, peeled,
   cored and chopped into 1cm/½in
   pieces, or canned pineapple in
   fruit juice, drained and chopped
4 tbsp raisins
4 eggs, beaten
80g/3oz/heaped ⅔ cup ground
   almonds
1 tsp bicarbonate of soda/baking soda
½ tsp baking powder
6 tbsp brown rice flour
80g/3oz/⅔ cup pumpkin seeds,
   finely chopped

1 Preheat the oven to 180°C/350°F/Gas 4 and grease a 20cm/8in loose-bottomed baking pan with oil.
2 Put the prunes and figs in a saucepan and add 150ml/5fl oz/scant ⅔ cup water. Bring to the boil over a medium heat, then reduce the heat to low and simmer for about 5 minutes, or until the water has been absorbed and the fruit is soft. Leave to cool for 10 minutes.
3 Put the pineapple into a mixing bowl and stir in the raisins and cooked fruit.
4 In a clean bowl, fold the eggs into the fruit mixture. Sift the ground almonds, bicarbonate of soda/baking soda, baking powder and flour into the mixture, add the pumpkin seeds and fold together. Pour the mixture into the baking pan and bake for 40 minutes, or until golden. Leave to cool for 5 minutes, then turn out onto a wire rack and leave to cool completely before serving.

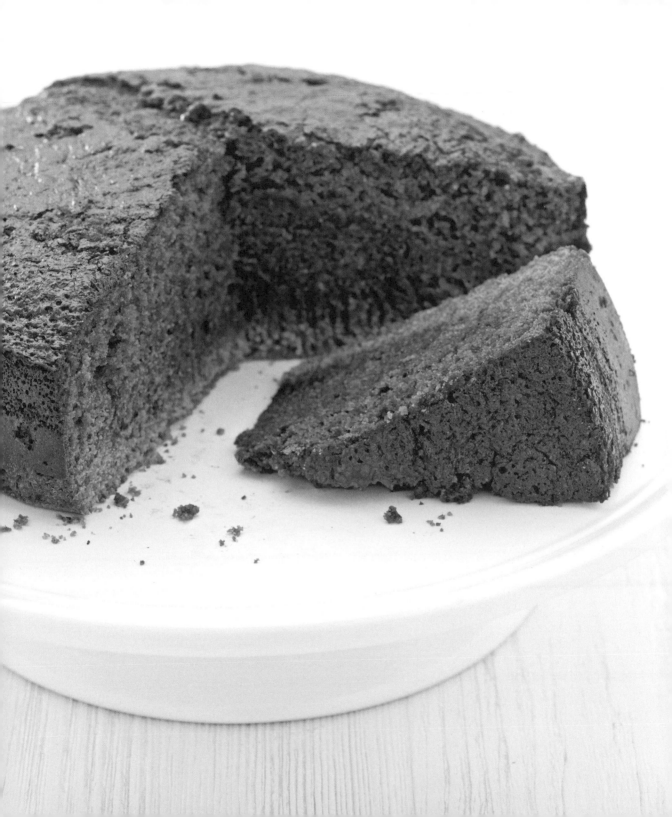

Phyto Fix Bars

sunflower oil, for greasing
50g/1¾oz/⅓ cup sesame seeds
100g/3½oz/⅔ cup flaxseeds
50g/1¾oz/½ cup sunflower seeds
50g/1¾oz/½ cup pumpkin seeds
100g/3½oz/heaped ¾ cup dried
   vine fruits, such as raisins,
   sultanas/golden raisins or currants
50g/1¾oz/scant ⅓ cup
   unsulphured dried apricots,
   chopped
75g/3oz soy protein isolate or soy
   protein powder
100g/3½oz/6 cups puffed rice
2 tsp mixed/apple pie spice
2 tsp ground ginger (optional)
100g/3½oz date syrup
50g/1¾oz ginger syrup or brown
   rice malt
150ml/5fl oz/scant ⅔ cup
   soy milk

1 Preheat the oven to 180°C/350°F/Gas 4 and grease a 30 x 20 x 2.5 cm/
  12 x 8 x 1in baking pan with sunflower oil.

2 Put all the dry ingredients in a large mixing bowl and mix. Pour in the syrups
  and soy milk and mix thoroughly. Spoon the mixture into the pan and smooth
  the surface with a palette knife/metal spatula or the back of a spoon.

3 Bake for 20 minutes, or until golden. Leave to cool for 5 minutes, then cut
  into 8 bars. Cool completely before serving.

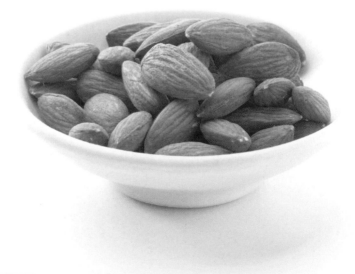

Chewy Fruit Bars

100ml/3½fl oz/scant ½ cup orange
  juice
100g/3½oz/heaped ½ cup
  unsulphured dried apricots,
  chopped
1 tsp grated orange zest
50g/1¾oz/⅓ cup almonds,
  chopped
50g/1¾oz/½ cup desiccated/dried
  shredded coconut, plus extra
  for sprinkling
50g/1¾oz/3 cups puffed rice
100g/3½oz/1 cup ground almonds
4 tbsp clear honey
50g/1¾oz/scant ½ cup dried fruit,
  such as raisins, apple or peach,
  chopped
toasted flaked/sliced almonds,
  for sprinkling

1 Preheat the oven to 180°C/350°F/Gas 4 and line a baking sheet with foil.
  Pour the orange juice into a medium-size saucepan and add the apricots and
  orange zest. Bring to the boil over a medium heat, then reduce the heat to
  low and simmer for 5 minutes, or until the liquid has been absorbed and the
  fruit is soft. Transfer to a large mixing bowl.

2 Put the chopped almonds and coconut on two separate baking sheets. Bake
  the almonds for 3–4 minutes until hot, and the coconut for 1 minute, or until
  lightly golden.

3 Add the puffed rice and ground almonds to the apricot mixture and stir well.
  Mix in the toasted coconut, toasted almonds, honey and dried fruit.

4 Using your hands, shape the mixture into a large ball and flatten. Transfer to
  the foil-lined baking sheet and, using your fingers, push the mixture to the
  edges of the pan evenly.

5 Sprinkle the mixture with a little coconut and the flaked/sliced almonds. Cut
  into 12 bars and chill in the refrigerator for about 3 hours to set. Store in a
  sealed container in the refrigerator and use within 1 week.

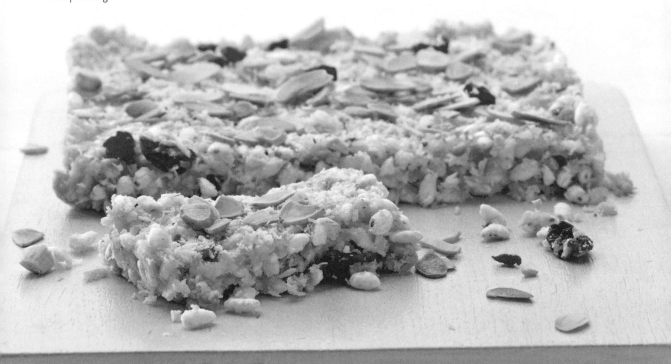

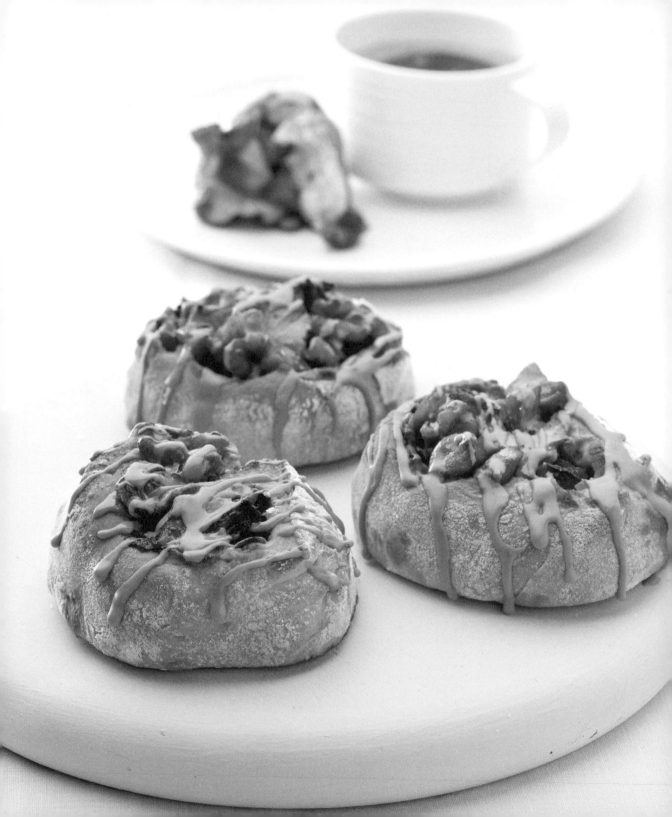

Apple & Walnut Coffee Rolls

70g/2½oz butter
350g/12oz tart green apples
   peeled, cored and diced
60g/2¼oz/½ cup chopped walnuts
½ tsp cinnamon
80g/2¾oz soft light brown sugar
350g/12oz/2¾ cups self-raising/
   self-rising flour, plus extra
   for dusting
250ml/9floz/1 cup soy milk

FROSTING
1 tsp coffee granules
80g/2¾oz/scant ⅔ cup icing/
   confectioners' sugar

1 Cut 30g/1oz of the butter into cubes and chill in the refrigerator.
2 Heat the remaining butter in a frying pan over a medium heat until melted. Add the apples and walnuts and cook, stirring occasionally, for 5 minutes, or until the apple softens. Add the cinnamon and sugar and cook, stirring frequently, for a further 6 minutes, until the sugar caramelizes. Remove from the heat and leave to cool for 5 minutes.
3 Sift the flour into a large mixing bowl and add the chilled butter. Using your fingertips, rub in the butter until the mixture resembles fine breadcrumbs. Make a well in the middle and pour in the soy milk. Using a round-bladed knife in a cutting action, mix the soy milk into the mixture to form a stiff dough. Press the dough into a ball with your hands, adding a little more flour if the dough is sticky. Cover with cling film/plastic wrap and chill in the refrigerator for 30 minutes.
4 Preheat the oven to 200°C/400°F/Gas 6 and line a baking sheet with baking parchment. Put the dough on a lightly floured surface and press it into a 20 x 30cm/8 x 12in rectangle. Spread the apple mixture over the dough, then take the long side of the dough and roll it up to enclose the filling. Put the roll seam-side down on a chopping board and cut into 8 equal-size pieces. Put these cut-side up on the baking sheet and bake for 20 minutes, or until golden brown. Remove from the sheet and leave to cool on a wire rack.
5 To make the frosting, put the coffee granules in a small bowl and add 1 tablespoon hot water. Mix well, then quickly stir in the icing/confectioners' sugar until the mixture is smooth. Drizzle the frosting over the rolls with a spoon and leave to set for 30 minutes, then serve.

Apple Bread Rolls

soy margarine, for greasing
100g/3¾oz tofu
100g/3¾oz grated apple
150ml/5fl oz/scant ⅔ cup
    unsweetened soy milk
2 eggs
50g/1¾oz/scant ½ cup potato flour
50g/1¾oz/scant ½ cup rice flour
50g/1¾oz/heaped ½ cup soy flour
50g/1¾oz/scant ½ cup cornmeal
1 tsp bicarbonate of soda/baking
    soda
½ tsp cream of tartar
¼ tsp tartaric acid
1 tbsp olive oil
1 tsp golden caster/superfine sugar

1 Preheat the oven to 220°C/425°F/Gas 7 and grease a 12-hole muffin pan with soy margarine.

2 Using a whisk, beat the tofu, apple, milk and eggs until smooth, and set aside.

3 Sift the flours, cornmeal, bicarbonate of soda/baking soda, cream of tartar and tartaric acid into a large mixing bowl and mix in the olive oil and sugar. Fold in the tofu mixture, making sure not to overmix or leave to stand, otherwise the batter will become too heavy.

4 Spoon the batter into the muffin pan and bake for 12–15 minutes, or until golden. Leave to cool for 5 minutes, then transfer to a wire rack to cool completely. Serve warm with sweet or savoury dishes.

Pictured right

VARIATION *Try 50g/1¾oz grated carrot instead of the tofu.*

Sussex Soy Bread

sunflower oil, for greasing
75g/2½oz/¾ cup soy flour
75g/2½oz/½ cup maize flour
150g/5½oz/heaped ¾ cup
    rice flour
2 tbsp soft light brown sugar
2 tbsp Phyto Sprinkle
    (see page 71)
1½ tsp fast-action dried yeast
2 heaped tsp baking powder
3 tbsp walnut oil
3 eggs
275ml/9½fl oz/1 cup unsweetened
    soy milk

1 Preheat the oven to 180°C/350°F/Gas 4 and grease a 900g/2lb loaf pan with sunflower oil. Sift the flours into the bowl of a food processor and add the sugar, Phyto Sprinkle, yeast and baking powder. Pour in the oil and blend thoroughly. Add the eggs, soy milk and 1 tablespoon cold water and blend until smooth.

2 Spoon the mixture into the loaf pan and bake for 50 minutes, or until golden brown. Leave to cool for 5 minutes, then turn out onto a wire rack. Leave to cool completely and then serve.

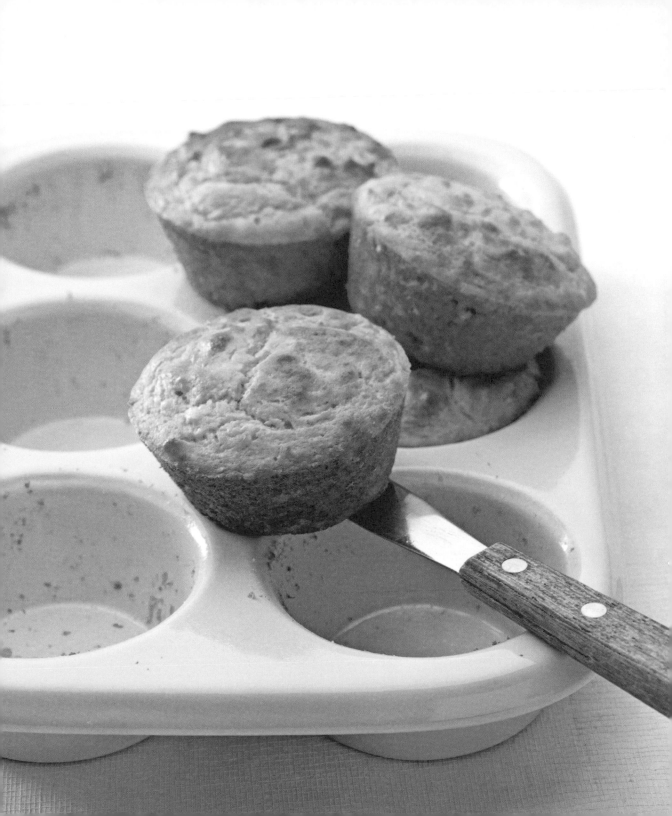

Quick & Easy Flat Bread

100g/4oz tofu
1 egg
150ml/5fl oz/scant ⅔ cup
   unsweetened soy milk
150g/5½oz/heaped ¾ cup rice
   flour
50g/1¾oz/scant ½ cup maize flour
25g/1oz/¼ cup soy flour
1 tsp bicarbonate of soda/
   baking soda
1 tsp cream of tartar
½ tsp tartaric acid
1 tsp golden caster/superfine sugar
1 tbsp soy oil

1 Preheat the oven to 220°C/425°F/Gas 7 and line a 25cm/10in square baking sheet with baking parchment. Put the tofu and egg in a blender or food processor and add the soy milk. Blend until smooth.

2 Sift the flours into a bowl and add the bicarbonate of soda/baking soda, cream of tartar, tartaric acid and sugar, then pour in the soy oil. Mix thoroughly and fold in the tofu mixture, making sure you do not overmix or leave to stand, otherwise the dough will become too heavy.

3 Spoon onto the baking tray and spread the mixture evenly with a palette knife/metal spatula or the back of a spoon.

4 Bake for 35 minutes, or until lightly golden. Leave to cool for 5 minutes, then turn out onto a wire rack. Serve warm.

Phyto Fruit Loaf

140g/5oz/heaped 1½ cups soy flour
100g/3½oz/½ cup buckwheat flour
100g/3½oz/½ cup flaxseeds
100g/3½oz/1 cup ground almonds
50g/1¾oz/⅓ cup sesame seeds
50g/1¾oz/⅓ cup sunflower seeds
280g/10oz dried fruit
2 tbsp unrefined caster/superfine
   sugar
1 tsp ground nutmeg
1 tsp mixed/apple pie spice
1 tbsp cinnamon
5cm/2in piece of root ginger
2 tsp baking powder
800ml/28fl oz/scant 3½ cups
   soy milk
sunflower oil, for greasing
butter, cheese, peanut butter
   or sugar-free jam, to serve

1 Sift the flours into a large mixing bowl and stir in the remaining dry ingredients. Pour in the soy milk and stir thoroughly to create a dough. Cover with cling film/plastic wrap and leave to stand at room temperature for 1 hour.

2 Preheat the oven to 180°C/350°F/Gas 4 and grease a 900g/2lb loaf tin with sunflower oil. Spoon the mixture into the loaf pan and bake for about 1 hour and 15 minutes, or until firm on top and golden. Leave to cool for 5 minutes then turn out onto a wire rack. Leave to cool for a further 10 minutes if you want to serve the loaf warm, or leave to cool completely. Serve with butter, cheese, peanut butter or jam.

Seed Bread

sunflower oil, for greasing
150g/5½oz/heaped 1½ cups soy
    flour
150g/5½oz/heaped ¾ cup rice
    flour
75g/2½oz/heaped ⅓ cup potato
    flour
2 tsp cream of tartar
1 tsp bicarbonate of soda/
    baking soda
75g/3oz/heaped ½ cup
    sunflower seeds
50g/2oz/⅓ cup sesame seeds
50g/2oz/scant ⅓ cup flaxseeds
50g/2oz/⅓ cup caraway seeds
2 tsp clear honey
310ml/10¾fl oz/1¼ cups
    unsweetened soy milk

1 Preheat the oven to 180°C/350°F/Gas 4 and grease a 450g/1lb loaf pan with sunflower oil. Sift the flours, cream of tartar and bicarbonate of soda/ baking soda into a large mixing bowl. Add the seeds and stir thoroughly. In a small bowl, beat together the honey and soy milk and stir into the dry ingredients.

2 Spoon the mixture into the loaf pan and bake for 40–45 minutes, or until golden and the sides of the bread come away from the pan. Leave to cool for 5 minutes, then turn out onto a wire rack and leave to cool completely before serving.

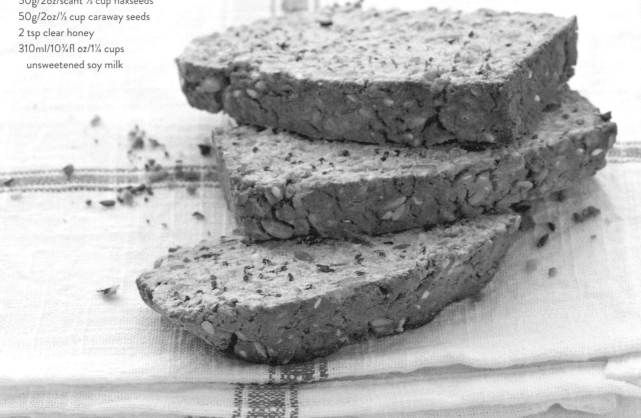

PHYTO-RICH MENU PLANS

Follow these menu plans for the first four weeks of your Natural Menopause Plan, then devise your own plans, making sure you consume 100mg of phytoestrogens over the course of each day (see page 27).

WEEK 1

DAY 1
Breakfast
Porridge/oatmeal made with soy milk and sprinkled with chopped banana, flaxseeds, almonds, sunflower seeds and pumpkin seeds
Lunch
Parsnip & Apple Soup (see page 86)
Oatcakes or French bread
1 piece of fresh fruit
Dinner
Spanish Chicken (see page 109)
Green beans
Baked potato
Dessert
Crème Caramel (see page 132)
Snacks
Unsulphured dried apricots
Phyto Fix Bar (see page 138)

DAY 2
Breakfast
Soy yogurt sprinkled with flaxseeds, chopped apple, sunflower seeds, pumpkin seeds and chopped pecan nuts
Lunch
Baked Potatoes with Spicy Soybeans (see page 94)
1 piece of fresh fruit
Dinner
Lamb's Liver with Orange (see page 115)
Roasted vegetables
Dessert
Prune and Tofu Dessert (see page 133)

Snacks
1 piece of fresh fruit
Phyto Fruit Loaf (see page 144)

DAY 3
Breakfast
Crunchy Almond Granola (see page 70) with soy milk and chopped pear
Lunch
Potato Skins with Broccoli and Tofu Filling (see page 96)
Salad
1 piece of fresh fruit
Soy yogurt
Dinner
Lamb & Aubergine Bake (see page 115)
Brown rice
Salad
Dessert
Apple & Tofu Cheesecake (see page 131)
Snacks
1 piece of fresh fruit
Mixed unsalted nuts

DAY 4
Breakfast
Banana Oat Crêpes (see page 68) with maple syrup, soy yogurt and chopped fresh fruit
Lunch
Brown Rice & Watercress Salad (see page 76)
1 piece of fresh fruit
Dinner
Salmon Steaks with Ginger (see page 107)

New potatoes
Green beans
Dessert
Crème Caramel (see page 132)
Snacks
1 piece of fresh fruit
Rice cakes with nut butter
Sunflower and pumpkin seeds

DAY 5
Breakfast
Scrambled Tofu (see page 67)
Lunch
Mushroom & Mint Soup (see page 90)
Seed Bread (see page 145) with soy cheese
1 piece of fresh fruit
Dinner
Lemon & Artichoke Risotto with Salmon & Asparagus (see page 100)
Dessert
Tofu Strawberry Dessert (see page 133)
Snacks
1 piece of fresh fruit
Oatcakes with pure fruit spread

DAY 6
Breakfast
Apple Bread Rolls (see page 142)
Creamy Banana & Date Shake (see page 66) with Phyto Sprinkle (see page 71)

Lunch
Turkish Tempeh on Pitta Bread (see page 94)
Dinner
Yogurt Roast Chicken (see page 112)
Baked potato
Salad
Dessert
Pineapple Cake (see page 136)
Snacks
1 piece of fresh fruit
Chewy Fruit Bar (see page 139)

DAY 7
Breakfast
Phyto Muesli (see page 71) with soy milk and chopped pear
Lunch
Sussex Soy Bread (see page 142) with soy cheese
Apple, Celery & Beetroot Salad (see page 84)
Dinner
Tuna & Fennel Pasta Bake (see page 106)
Dessert
Ginger Fruit Salad (see page 135) with soy cream
Snacks
Apple & Walnut Coffee Rolls (see page 141)
Banana Shake (see page 64)

WEEK 2

DAY 1
Breakfast
Porridge with Spiced Fruit
  Compôte (see page 72)
  with soy milk, flaxseeds and
  chopped pear
Lunch
Rosemary Arancini (see page 95)
Salad
1 piece of fresh fruit and soy
  yogurt
Dinner
Individual Moussakas
  (see page 114)
Salad
Dessert
Banana & Rice Pudding
  (see page 132)
Snacks
Unsulphured dried apricots
Phyto Fix Bar (see page 138)

DAY 2
Breakfast
Crunchy Almond Granola
  (see page 70) with soy
  milk and chopped apple
Lunch
Bean Tacos (see page 98)
Salad
1 piece of fresh fruit
Dinner
Mackerel with Lemon & Ginger
  (see page 104)
New potatoes
Salad
Dessert
Banana & Raspberry Bread
  (see page 135) with soy
  cream cheese and honey

Snacks
1 piece of fresh fruit
Fruit & Nut Shake (see page 67)

DAY 3
Breakfast
Puffed rice cereal with soy
  milk sprinkled with chopped
  banana, pecan nuts and
  Phyto Sprinkle (see page 71)
Lunch
Carrot & Apricot Pâté (see
  page 91)
Oatcakes
Summer Salad (see page 79)
Dinner
Yogurt Roast Chicken (see
  page 112)
Roast potatoes
Carrots
Cabbage
Dessert
Raspberry & Tofu Brulée (see
  page 131)
Snacks
1 piece of fresh fruit
Ginger Cake (see page 136)

DAY 4
Breakfast
Chilli & Corn Fritters with
  Scrambled Eggs (see page 75)
Lunch
Endive, Fruit & Nut Salad
  (see page 82)
Seed Bread (see page 145)
  with soy cheese

Dinner
Tofu & Vegetable Rice (see
  page 121)
Dessert
Apple & Tofu Cheesecake (see
  page 131)
Snacks
1 piece of fresh fruit
Rhubarb & Blueberry Smoothie
  (see page 64)

DAY 5
Breakfast
Cornflakes with soy milk,
  chopped banana, almonds and
  Phyto Sprinkle (see page 71)
Lunch
Lentil Scotch Eggs with Tofu
  Dressing (see page 85)
Salad
1 piece of fresh fruit
Dinner
Mustard Cod Crêpes (see page
  102)
Dessert
Pineapple Cake (see page 136)
Snacks
1 piece of fresh fruit
Phyto Fix Bar (see page 138)

DAY 6
Breakfast
Scrambled Tofu (see page 67)
  with tomato and mushrooms
  on rye bread
Lunch
Watercress Soup (see page 86)

Seed Bread (see page 145) with
  soy cheese
1 piece of fresh fruit
Dinner
Creamy Chicken Curry (see
  page 109)
Rice
Poppadam
Dessert
Prune and Tofu Dessert (see
  page 133)
Snacks
Phyto Fruit Loaf (see page 144)
Mixed nuts

DAY 7
Breakfast
1 piece of fresh fruit
Creamy Banana & Date Shake
  (see page 66) with Phyto
  Sprinkle (see page 71)
Lunch
Hummus (see page 91)
Quick & Easy Flat Bread (see
  page 144)
Bean Salad (see page 83)
Dinner
Poached Halibut with Parsley
  Sauce (see page 104)
New potatoes
Green beans
Dessert
Crème Caramel (see page 132)
Snacks
1 piece of fresh fruit
Apple & Walnut Coffee Rolls
  (see page 141)

WEEK 3

DAY 1
Breakfast
Soy & Rice Crêpes (see page 69) with fresh berries
Lunch
Corn Chowder with Garlic Prawns (see page 89)
Rye bread
1 piece of fresh fruit
Soy yogurt
Dinner
Indonesian Tofu Kebabs with Satay Sauce (see page 118)
Rice
Green beans
Dessert
Banana & Rice Pudding (see page 132)
Snacks
Fruit & Nut Shake (see page 67)
Sunflower seeds and pumpkin seeds

DAY 2
Breakfast
Phyto Muesli (see page 71) with soy milk and chopped banana
Lunch
Niçoise Salad with Soy Dressing (see page 80)
1 piece of fresh fruit
Dinner
Lasagne (see page 119)
Salad
Dessert
Tofu Strawberry Dessert (see page 133)
Snacks
Seed Bread (see page 145), toasted, with pure fruit spread
Unsulphured dried apricots

DAY 3
Breakfast
Porridge with Spiced Fruit Compôte (see page 72) with Phyto Sprinkle (see page 71) and soy milk
Lunch
Edamame Bean & Vegetable Soup (see page 90)
Seed Bread (see page 145) with soy cheese
Dinner
Mushroom & Spinach Quiche (see page 123)
Salad
Dessert
Ginger Cake (see page 136) with soy yogurt
Snacks
1 piece of fresh fruit
Oatcakes with nut butter

DAY 4
Breakfast
Soy yogurt sprinkled with almonds and flaxseeds
Apple & Walnut Coffee Rolls (see page 141)
Lunch
Spanish Omelette (see page 98)
Salad
1 piece of fresh fruit
Dinner
Sweet Soy Sauce Fish with Spinach (see page 106)
Green salad
Dessert
Ginger Fruit Salad (see page 135)
Snacks
Phyto Fix Bar (see page 138)
Mixed unsalted nuts

DAY 5
Breakfast
Scrambled Tofu (see page 67) with tomato and mushrooms on rye bread
Lunch
Orange & Avocado Salad (see page 83)
Seed Bread (see page 145) with soy cheese
1 piece of fresh fruit
Dinner
Thai Green Curry (see page 110)
Jasmine rice
Dessert
Soy yogurt sprinkled with sunflower seeds and pumpkin seeds
Snacks
Banana & Raspberry Bread (see page 135)
Rhubarb & Blueberry Smoothie (see page 64)

DAY 6
Breakfast
Crunchy Almond Granola (see page 70) with soy milk and chopped pear
Lunch
Tofu, Bean & Herb Stir-Fry (see page 92)
Rice
Dinner
Falafel with Sesame Yogurt Dressing (see page 127)
Pitta bread
Salad
Dessert
Raspberry & Tofu Brûlée (see page 131)
Snacks
1 piece of fresh fruit
Rice cakes with nut butter
Sunflower and pumpkin seeds

DAY 7
Breakfast
Soy & Buckwheat Crêpes (see page 68)
Lunch
Tempeh with Pak Choi & Noodles (see page 92)
Dinner
Pork with Orange & Herb Sauce (see page 116)
New potatoes
Broccoli
Green beans
Dessert
Strawberry Soufflé Pancakes (see page 128)
Soy cream
Snacks
1 piece of fresh fruit
Chewy Fruit Bar (see page 139)

WEEK 4

DAY 1

Breakfast
Phyto Muesli (see page 71) with soy milk and chopped pear

Lunch
Chicken Noodle Soup (see page 89)
Rye bread
1 piece of fresh fruit
Soy yogurt

Dinner
Spanish Omelette Bake (see page 123)
Salad

Dessert
Pineapple Cake (see page 136)

Snacks
1 piece of fresh fruit
Honey & Cinnamon Soy Milk (see page 66)
Sunflower and pumpkin seeds

DAY 2

Breakfast
Soy yogurt sprinkled with chopped apple, flaxseeds, sunflower seeds, pumpkin seeds and chopped pecan nuts

Lunch
Refried Soybeans (see page 97)
Taco shells
1 piece of fresh fruit

Dinner
Beef Stir-Fry with Apricots and Walnuts (see page 112)
Rice
Courgettes/zucchini

Dessert
Prune & Tofu Dessert (see page 133)

Snacks
Fruit & Nut Shake (see page 67)
1 piece of fresh fruit

DAY 3

Breakfast
Banana Oat Crêpes (see page 68) with maple syrup, soy yogurt and chopped fresh fruit

Lunch
Hummus (see page 91) with crudités
Oatcakes
1 piece of fresh fruit

Dinner
Tofu "Meatballs" (see page 120)
Rice
Broccoli
Courgettes/zucchini

Dessert
Ginger Cake (see page 136) with soy yogurt

Snacks
Seed Bread (see page 145), toasted, with pure fruit spread
Unsulphured dried apricots

DAY 4

Breakfast
Rice cakes with pure fruit spread
Soy yogurt with chopped fresh fruit and flaxseeds

Lunch
Apple & Nut Salad (see page 82)
Seed Bread (see page 145) with soy cheese

Dinner
Spinach & Cheese Soufflé (see page 124)
Salad

Dessert
Apple & Tofu Cheesecake (see page 131)

Snacks
1 piece of fresh fruit
Oatcakes with nut butter

DAY 5

Breakfast
Porridge/oatmeal made with soy milk and sprinkled with unsulphured dried apricots, flaxseeds and almonds

Lunch
Oriental Rice Salad (see page 79)
1 piece of fresh fruit
Soy yogurt

Dinner
Poached Fish Balls (see page 103)
Rice
Broccoli
Green beans

Dessert
Tofu Strawberry Dessert (see page 133)

Snacks
Seed Bread (see page 145), toasted, with pure fruit spread
Mixed unsalted nuts

DAY 6

Breakfast
Crunchy Almond Granola (see page 70) with soy milk and chopped banana

Lunch
Coleslaw (see page 82)
Baked potato
Fruit & Nut Shake (see page 67)

Dinner
Red Lentil & Coconut Cream (see page 120)
Rice
Courgettes/zucchini

Dessert
Ginger Fruit Salad (see page 135) with soy cream

Snacks
1 piece of fresh fruit
Banana & Raspberry Bread (see page 135)

DAY 7

Breakfast
Soy yogurt sprinkled with chopped banana, sunflower seeds, flaxseeds, pumpkin seeds and chopped pecan nuts

Lunch
Corn Chowder with Garlic Prawns (see page 89)
Rye bread
1 piece of fresh fruit
Soy yogurt

Dinner
Noodles in Spicy Sesame Sauce (see page 116)
Broccoli
Green beans

Dessert
Raspberry & Tofu Brûlée (see page 131)

Snacks
1 piece of fresh fruit
Rice cakes with nut butter
Sunflower and pumpkin seeds

NUTRIENT CONTENT OF FOODS

Use these tables to guide you in your daily food choices. Foods are raw unless otherwise stated.

Vitamin A – retinol

Micrograms per 100g/3½oz

Skimmed/skim milk 1
Semi-skimmed/2% milk 21
Herring, grilled/broiled 49
Whole milk 52
Porridge/oatmeal, made
   with milk 56
Cheddar cheese 325
Margarine 800
Butter 815
Lamb's liver, cooked 15,000

Vitamin B1 – thiamin

Micrograms per 100g/3½oz

Peaches 0.02
Cottage cheese 0.02
Cox's apple 0.03
Full-fat/whole milk 0.04
Skimmed/skim milk 0.04
Semi-skimmed/2% milk 0.04
Cheddar cheese 0.04
Bananas 0.04
White grapes 0.04
French/thin green beans,
   cooked 0.04
Low-fat yogurt 0.05
Cantaloupe melon 0.05
Tomato 0.06
Green peppers 0.07
Egg, boiled 0.08
Chicken, roast 0.08
Cod, grilled/broiled 0.08
Haddock, steamed 0.08

Turkey, roast 0.09
Mackerel, cooked 0.09
Savoy cabbage, boiled 0.10
Oranges 0.1
Brussels sprouts, boiled 0.1
Potatoes, new, boiled 0.11
Soybeans, boiled 0.12
Red peppers 0.12
Lentils, boiled 0.14
Salmon, steamed 0.2
Corn 0.2
White spaghetti, boiled 0.21
Almonds 0.24
White self-raising/self-rising
   flour 0.3
Plaice/flounder, steamed 0.3
Bacon, cooked 0.35
Walnuts 0.4
Wholemeal/whole-wheat
   flour 0.47
Lamb's kidney, cooked 0.49
Brazil nuts 1
Cornflakes 1
Crisped rice cereal 1
Wheatgerm 2.01

Vitamin B2 – riboflavin

Micrograms per 100g/3½oz

Cabbage, boiled 0.01
Potatoes, boiled 0.01
Brown rice, boiled 0.02
Pear 0.03
Wholemeal spaghetti, cooked
   0.03

White self-raising/self-rising
   flour 0.03
Orange 0.04
Spinach, cooked 0.05
Baked beans 0.06
Banana 0.06
White bread 0.06
Green peppers 0.08
Lentils, boiled 0.08
Soybeans, boiled 0.09
Wholemeal/whole-wheat bread
   0.09
Wholemeal/whole-wheat flour
   0.09
Peanuts 0.1
Salmon, baked 0.11
Red peppers 0.15
Full-fat/whole milk 0.17
Avocado 0.18
Herring, grilled/broiled 0.18
Semi-skimmed/2% milk 0.18
Chicken, roast 0.19
Turkey, roast 0.21
Cottage cheese 0.26
Soy flour 0.31
Prawns/shrimp, boiled 0.34
Egg, boiled 0.35
Topside of beef, cooked 0.35
Leg of lamb, cooked 0.38
Cheddar cheese 0.4
Muesli 0.7
Almonds 0.75
Cornflakes 1.5
Crisped rice cereal 1.5

Vitamin B3 – niacin

Micrograms per 100g/3½oz

Egg, boiled 0.07
Cheddar cheese 0.07
Full-fat/whole milk 0.08
Skimmed/skim milk 0.09
Semi-skimmed/2% milk 0.09
Cottage cheese 0.13
Cox's apple 0.2
Cabbage, boiled 0.3
Orange 0.4
Baked beans 0.5
Potatoes, boiled 0.5
Soybeans, boiled 0.5
Lentils, boiled 0.6
Banana 0.7
Tomato 1
Avocado 1.1
Green peppers 1.1
Brown rice 1.3
Wholemeal/whole-wheat
   spaghetti, boiled 1.3
White self-raising/self-rising
   flour 1.5
Cod, grilled/broiled 1.7
White bread 1.7
Soy flour 2
Red peppers 2.2
Almonds 3.1
Herring, grilled/broiled 4
Wholemeal/whole-wheat bread
   4.1
Wholemeal/whole-wheat flour
   5.7

Muesli 6.5

Topside of beef, cooked 6.5

Leg of lamb, cooked 6.6

Salmon, baked 7

Chicken, roast 8.2

Turkey, roast 8.5

Prawns/shrimps, boiled 9.5

Peanuts 13.8

Crisped rice cereal 16

Cornflakes 16

Vitamin B6 – pyridoxine

Micrograms per 100g/3½oz

Carrots 0.05

Full-fat/whole milk 0.06

Skimmed/skim milk 0.06

Semi-skimmed/2% milk 0.06

Satsuma 0.07

White bread 0.07

White rice 0.07

Cabbage, boiled 0.08

Cottage cheese 0.08

Cox's apple 0.08

Wholemeal/whole-wheat pasta, cooked 0.08

Peas, frozen 0.09

Spinach, boiled 0.09

Cheddar cheese 0.1

Orange 0.1

Broccoli, boiled 0.11

Baked beans 0.12

Egg, boiled 0.12

Red kidney beans, boiled 0.12

Wholemeal/whole-wheat bread 0.12

Tomatoes 0.14

Almonds 0.15

Cauliflower, boiled 0.15

Brussels sprouts, boiled 0.19

Sweetcorn, boiled 0.21

Leg of lamb, cooked 0.22

Grapefruit juice 0.23

Chicken, roast 0.26

Lentils, boiled 0.28

Banana 0.29

Brazil nuts 0.31

Potatoes, boiled 0.32

Turkey, roast 0.33

Herring, grilled/broiled 0.33

Topside of beef, cooked 0.33

Avocado 0.36

Cod, grilled/broiled 0.38

Salmon, baked 0.57

Soy flour 0.57

Hazelnuts 0.59

Peanuts 0.59

Walnuts 0.67

Muesli 1.6

Cornflakes 1.8

Crisped rice cereal 1.8

Vitamin B12 – cyanocobalamine

Micrograms per 100g/3½oz

Tempeh 0.1

Miso 0.2

Mycoprotein 0.3

Full-fat/whole milk 0.4

Skimmed/skim milk 0.4

Semi-skimmed/2% milk 0.4

Yeast extract 0.5

Cottage cheese 0.7

Choux buns 1

Eggs, boiled 1

Eggs, poached 1

Halibut, steamed 1

Lobster, boiled 1

Sponge cake 1

Turkey, white meat 1

Waffles 1

Cheddar cheese 1.2

Eggs, scrambled 1.2

Squid 1.3

Eggs, fried 1.6

Shrimps, boiled 1.8

Parmesan cheese 1.9

Beef, lean, cooked 2

Cod, baked 2

Cornflakes 2

Pork, cooked 2

Crisped rice cereal 2

Steak, lean, grilled/broiled 2

Edam cheese 2.1

Eggs, whole, battery, boiled 2.4

Milk, dried, whole 2.4

Milk, dried, skimmed/skim 2.6

Eggs, whole, free-range, boiled 2.7

Kambu seaweed 2.8

Squid, frozen, cooked 2.9

Taramasalata 2.9

Duck, roasted 3

Turkey, dark meat, roasted 3

Grapenuts 5

Tuna, canned in oil 5

Herring, cooked 6

Herring roe, fried 6

Salmon, steamed 6

Beef extract 8.3

Mackerel, fried 10

Rabbit, stewed 10

Cod's roe, fried 11

Oysters 15

Nori seaweed 27.5

Sardines, canned in oil 28

Lamb's kidney, fried 79

Folate/Folic Acid

Micrograms per 100g/3½oz

Cox's apple 4

Leg of lamb, cooked 4

Full-fat/whole milk 6

Skimmed/skim milk 6

Semi-skimmed/2% milk 6

Porridge/oatmeal with low-fat milk 7

Turnip, baked 8

Cucumber 9

Herring, grilled/broiled 10

Chicken, roast 10

Avocado 11

Cod, grilled/broiled 12

Banana 14

Turkey, roast 15

Carrots 17

Sweet potato, baked 17

Tomatoes 17

Topside of beef, cooked 17

Swede/rutabaga, boiled 18

Strawberries 20

Brazil nuts 21

Red peppers 21

Green peppers 23

Rye bread 24

Dates, fresh 25

New potatoes, boiled 25

Grapefruit 26

Oatcakes 26

Cottage cheese 27

Salmon, baked 29

Cabbage, boiled 29

Onions, boiled 29

White bread 29

Orange 31

Baked beans 33

Cheddar cheese 33

Clementines 33

Raspberries 33

Satsuma 33

Blackberries 34

Rye crispbread 35

Potato, baked in skin 36

Radish 38

Egg, boiled 39

Wholemeal/whole-wheat bread 39

Red kidney beans, boiled 42

Potato, baked 44

Peas, frozen 47

Almonds 48

Parsnips, boiled 48

Cauliflower 51

Green beans, boiled 57

Broccoli 64

Walnuts 66

Artichoke, boiled 68

Hazelnuts 72

Spinach, boiled 90

Brussels sprouts 110

Peanuts 110

Muesli 140

Sweetcorn, boiled 150

Asparagus 155

Chickpeas 180

Lamb's liver, fried 240

Cornflakes 250

Crisped rice cereal 250

Calf's liver, fried 320

Vitamin C
Micrograms per 100g/3½oz

Full-fat/whole milk 1

Skimmed/skim milk 1

Red kidney beans, boiled 1

Carrots 2

Cucumber 2

Muesli with dried fruit 2

Apricots 6

Avocado 6

Pear 6

Potato, boiled 6

Spinach, boiled 8

Cox's apple 9

Turnip 10

Banana 11

Peas, frozen 12

Lamb's liver, fried 12

Pineapple 12

Dried skimmed/skim milk 13

Gooseberries, boiled 14

Dates 14

Melon 17

Tomatoes 17

Cabbage, boiled 20

Canteloupe melon 26

Cauliflower 27

Satsuma 27

Peach 31

Raspberries 32

Bran flakes 35

Grapefruit 36

Mangoes 37

Nectarine 37

Kumquats 39

Broccoli, boiled 44

Lychees 45

Unsweetened apple juice 49

Orange 54

Kiwi fruit 59

Brussels sprouts 60

Strawberries 77

Blackcurrants 115

Vitamin D
Micrograms per 100g/3½oz

Skimmed/skim milk 0.01

Full-fat/whole milk 0.03

Fromage frais/blanc 0.05

Cheddar cheese 0.26

Cornflakes 2.8

Crisped rice cereal 2.8

Margarine 8

Vitamin E
Micrograms per 100g/3½oz

Semi-skimmed/2% milk 0.03

Potatoes, boiled 0.06

Cucumber 0.07

Cottage cheese 0.08

Full-fat/whole milk 0.09

Cabbage, boiled 0.1

Leg of lamb, cooked 0.1

Cauliflower, boiled 0.11

Chicken, roast 0.11

Peas, frozen 0.18

Red kidney beans, boiled 0.2

Wholemeal/whole-wheat bread 0.2

Orange 0.24

Topside of beef, cooked 0.26

Banana 0.27

Brown rice, boiled 0.3

Herring, grilled/broiled 0.3

Lamb's liver, fried 0.32

Baked beans 0.36

Cornflakes 0.4

Pear 0.5

Cheddar cheese 0.53

Carrots 0.56

Lettuce 0.57

Cox's apple 0.59

Cod, grilled/broiled 0.59

Crisped rice cereal 0.6

Plums 0.61

Unsweetened orange juice 0.68

Leeks, boiled 0.78

Sweetcorn, boiled 0.88

Brussels sprouts 0.9

Broccoli 1.1

Egg, boiled 1.11

Tomato 1.22

Watercress 1.46

Parsley 1.7

Spinach, boiled 1.71

Olives 1.99

Butter 2

Onions, dried raw 2.69

Mushrooms, fried 2.84

Avocado 3.2

Muesli 3.2

Walnuts 3.85

Peanut butter 4.99
Olive oil 5.1
Sweet potato, baked 5.96
Brazil nuts 7.18
Peanuts 10.09
Pine nuts 13.65
Rapeseed/canola oil 18.4
Almonds 23.96
Hazelnuts 24.98
Sunflower oil 48.7

Calcium

Micrograms per 100g/3½oz

Cox's apple 4
Brown rice, boiled 4
Potatoes, boiled 5
Banana 6
Topside of beef, cooked 6
White pasta, boiled 7
Tomato 7
Leg of lamb, cooked 8
Red peppers 8
Chicken, roast 9
Turkey, roast 9
Avocado 11
Pear 11
Butter 15
Cornflakes 15
White rice, boiled 18
Cod, grilled/broiled 22
Lentils, boiled 22
Baked salmon 29
Green peppers 30
Young carrots 30
Herring, grilled/broiled 33
Wholemeal/whole-wheat flour 38
Turnips, baked 45
Orange 47

Baked beans 48
Wholemeal/whole-wheat bread 54
Egg, boiled 57
Peanuts 60
Cottage cheese 73
Soybeans, boiled 83
White bread 100
Full-fat/whole milk 115
Muesli 120
Skimmed/skim milk 120
Semi-skimmed/2% milk 120
Prawns/shrimps, boiled 150
Spinach, boiled 150
Brazil nuts 70
Yogurt, low-fat, plain 190
Soy flour 210
Almonds 240.0
White self-raising/self-rising flour 450
Sardines 550
Sprats, fried 710
Cheddar cheese 720
Whitebait, fried 860

Chromium

Micrograms per 100g/3½oz

Fruit juices 47
Liver, cooked 55
Hard cheese 56
Beef, cooked 57
Brewer's yeast 117
Molasses 121
Egg yolk, cooked 183

Iron

Micrograms per 100g/3½oz

Semi-skimmed/2% milk 0.05
Skimmed/skim milk 0.06

Full-fat/whole milk 0.06
Cottage cheese 0.1
Orange 0.1
Cox's apple 0.2
Pear 0.2
White rice, boiled 0.2
Banana 0.3
Cabbage, boiled 0.3
Cheddar cheese 0.3
Avocado 0.4
Cod, grilled/broiled 0.4
Potatoes, boiled 0.4
Young carrots, boiled 0.4
Brown rice, boiled 0.5
Tomato 0.5
White pasta, boiled 0.5
Salmon, baked 0.8
Chicken, roast 0.8
Turkey, roast 0.9
Herring, grilled/broiled 1
Red peppers 1
Prawns/shrimps, boiled 1.1
Green peppers 1.2
Baked beans 1.4
Wholemeal/whole-wheat spaghetti, cooked 1.4
White bread 1.6
Spinach, boiled 1.7
Egg, boiled 1.9
White self-raising/self-rising flour 2
Brazil nuts 2.5
Peanuts 2.5
Leg of lamb, cooked 2.7
Wholemeal/whole-wheat bread 2.7
Topside of beef, cooked 2.8
Almonds 3
Soybeans, boiled 3

Lentils, boiled 3.5
Wholemeal/whole-wheat flour 3.9
Muesli 5.6
Cornflakes 6.7
Crisped rice cereal 6.7
Soy flour 6.9

Magnesium

Micrograms per 100g/3½oz

Butter 2
Cox's apple 6
Turnip, baked 6
Young carrots 6
Tomato 7
Cottage cheese 9
Orange 10
Full-fat/whole milk 11
White rice, boiled 11
Semi-skimmed/2% milk 11
Skimmed/skim milk 12
Egg, boiled 12
Cornflakes 14
Potatoes, boiled 14
Red peppers 14
White pasta, boiled 15
Wholemeal/whole-wheat spaghetti, cooked 15
White self-raising/self-rising flour 20
Green peppers 24
Chicken, roast 24
Topside of beef, cooked 24
White bread 24
Avocado 25
Cheddar cheese 25
Cod, grilled/broiled 26
Turkey, roast 27
Leg of lamb, cooked 28

Salmon, baked 29
Baked beans 31
Spinach, boiled 31
Herring, grilled/broiled 32
Banana 34
Lentils, boiled 34
Prawns/shrimp, boiled 42
Wholemeal/whole-wheat
    spaghetti, cooked 42
Brown rice, boiled 43
Soybeans, boiled 63
Wholemeal/whole-wheat
    bread 76
Muesli 85
Wholemeal/whole-wheat
    flour 120
Peanuts 210
Soy flour 240
Almonds 270
Brazil nuts 410

Selenium

Micrograms per 100g/3½oz
Full-fat/whole milk 1
Skimmed/skim milk 1
Baked beans 2
Cornflakes 2
Orange 2
Peanuts 3
Almonds 4
Cottage cheese 4

White rice 4
White self-raising/self-rising
    flour 4
Soybeans, boiled 5
Egg, boiled 11
Cheddar cheese 12
White bread 28
Wholemeal/whole-wheat bread
    35
Lentils, boiled 40
Wholemeal/whole-wheat flour
    53
Brazil nuts 1,900

Zinc

Micrograms per 100g/3½oz
Butter 0.1
Pear 0.1
Orange 0.1
Red peppers 0.1
Banana 0.2
Young carrots 0.2
Cornflakes 0.3
Potatoes, boiled 0.3
Avocado 0.4
Full-fat/whole milk 0.4
Skimmed/skim milk 0.4
Green peppers 0.4
Semi-skimmed/2% milk 0.4
Baked beans 0.5
Cod, grilled/broiled 0.5

Herring, grilled/broiled 0.5
White pasta, boiled 0.5
Tomatoes 0.5
Cottage cheese 0.6
Spinach, boiled 0.6
White bread 0.6
White self-raising/self-rising
    flour 0.6
Brown rice, boiled 0.7
White rice, boiled 0.7
Soybeans, boiled 0.9
Wholemeal/whole-wheat
    spaghetti, cooked 1.1
Egg, boiled 1.3
Lentils, boiled 1.4
Chicken, roast 1.5
Prawns/shrimps, boiled 1.6
Wholemeal/whole-wheat bread
    1.8
Cheddar cheese 2.3
Turkey, roast 2.4
Muesli 2.5
Wholemeal/whole-wheat flour
    2.9
Almonds 3.2
Peanuts 3.5
Brazil nuts 4.2
Leg of lamb, cooked 5.3
Topside of beef, cooked 5.5

Essential fatty acids

*Exact amounts of these fats are
hard to quantify. Good sources for
the two families of essential fatty
acids are listed below.*

**Omega-6 series essential
fatty acids**
Sunflower oil
Rapeseed/canola oil
Corn oil
Almonds
Walnuts
Brazil nuts
Sunflower seeds
Soy products including tofu

**Omega-3 series essential
fatty acids**
Mackerel
Herring
Salmon
Trout
Avocado
Walnuts
Walnut oil
Rapeseed/canola oil
Olive oil

REFERENCES

General

Dennerstein, L., Wood, C., Westmore, A., *Hysterectomy: New Options and Advances,* 2nd edition, Oxford University Press, 1999

Pizzorno, J.E., Murray, M.T., Joiner-Bey, H., (eds) *Textbook of Natural Medicine,* 2nd edition, Churchill Livingstone, 2007

Rees, M., Stephenson, J., Hope, S., Rozenberg, S., Santiago, P., *Management of the Menopause,* 5th edition, Oxford University Press, 2010

Stewart, M., *Cruising Through the Menopause,* Vermilion, 2000

Stewart, M., *Beat Menopause Naturally,* Natural Health Publications, London 2006

Stewart, M., *The Phyto Factor,* Vermilion, 2000

Menopause

Anderson, G.L., Limacher, M., Assaf, A.R., et al, Effects of conjugated equine estrogen in postmenopausal women with hysterectomy: the Women's Health Initiative randomized controlled trial. *JAMA* 2004; 291(14): 1701–12

Chiechi, L.M., Putignano, G., Guerra, V., et al, The effect of a soya rich diet on the vaginal epithelium in post menopause: a randomized double blind trial. *Maturitas* 2003; 45(4): 241–6

Helena Hachul, MD, PhD, et al, Isoflavones decrease insomnia in postmenopause.*The Journal of The North American Menopause Society* Vol. 18, No. 2, pp.1–7

Komesaroff, P.A., Black, C.V., Cable, V., Sudhir, K., Effects of wild yam extract on menopausal symptoms, lipids and sex hormones in healthy postmenopausal women. *Climacteric* 2001; 4(2): 144–50

Rossouw, J.E., Anderson, G.L., Prentice, R.L., (Division of Women's Health Initiative). Risks and benefits of estrogen plus progestin in healthy postmenopausal women: principal results from the Women's Health Initiative randomized controlled trial. *JAMA* 2002; 288(3): 321–33

Royal College of Obstetrics and Gynaecology. Scientific Advisory Committee Opinion Paper 6: Alternatives to HRT for management of symptoms of the menopause. RCOG, May 2006

Treatment of menopause-associated vasomotor symptoms: position statement of the North American Menopause Society, *Menopause* 2004; 11(1): 11–33

Wilcox G., Wahlqvist, M.L., Burger, H.G., Medley, G., Oestrogenic effects of plant foods in postmenopausal women. *BMJ* 1990; 301(6757); 905–6

Phytoestrogens

Adlercreutz, H., Hamalainen, E., Gorbach, S., Goldin, B., Dietary phytoestrogens and the menopause in Japan. *Lancet.* 1992; 339 (8803): 1233

Cutler, G.J., Nettleton, J.A., Ross, J.A., et al, Dietary flavonoid intake and risk of cancer in postmenopausal women: the Iowa Women's Health Study. *Int J Cancer*

Ferrari, A., Soy extract phytoestrogens with high dose of isoflavones for menopausal symptoms. *J Obstet Gynaecol Res* 2009; 35: 1083–90

Hall, W.L., Vafeiadou, K., Hallund, J., et al, Soya-isoflavone-enriched foods and inflammatory biomarkers of cardiovascular disease risk in postmenopausal women: interactions with genotype and equol production. *Am J Clin Nutr.* 2005; 82(6): 1260–1268

Hooper L., Ryder, J.J., Kurzer, M.S., et al, Effects of soy protein and isoflavones on circulating hormone concentrations in pre- and post-menopausal women: a systematic review and meta-analysis. *Hum. Reprod. Update* 2009;15:423-40.

Howes, L.G., Howes, J.B., Knight, D.C., Isoflavone therapy for menopausal flushes: a systematic review and meta-analysis. *Maturitas.* 2006; 55: 203–11

Kurzer, M.S., et al, Soya isoflavones decrease hot-flash frequency: a meta-analysis of studies examining soya protein, soya food, and soya isoflavones. Orlando, Florida: Fifth International Symposium on the Role of Soya in Preventing and Treating Chronic Disease, Sept 21–24, 2003

Setchell, K.D.R., Cole, S.J., Method of defining equol-producer status and its frequency among vegetarians. *J Nutr.* 2006; 136: 2188–93

Williamson-Hughes, P.S., Flickinger, B.D., Messina, M.J., Empie, M.W., Isoflavone supplements containing predominantly genistein reduce hot flash symptoms: a critical review of published studies. *Menopause.* 2006; 13: 831–9

Lignans

Franco, O.H., Burger, H., Lebrun, C.E., et al, Higher dietary intake of lignans is associated with better cognitive performance in postmenopausal women. *J Nutr.* 2005; 135(5): 1190–1195

Lemay, A., Dodin, S., Kadri, N., Jacques, H., Forest, J.C., Flaxseed dietary supplement versus hormone replacement therapy in hypercholesterolemic menopausal women. *Obstet Gynecol.* 2002; 100(3): 495–504

Sacks, F., Lichtenstein, A., Van Horn, L., et al, Soya protein, isoflavones and cardiovascular health: an American Heart Association Science Advisory for professionals from the Nutrition Committee. 504. *Circulation* 2006; 113(7): 1034–1044

Supplements

Atkinson, C., Warren, R.M., Sala E., et al, Red-clover-derived isoflavones and mammographic breast density: a double-blind, randomized, placebo-controlled trial. *Breast Cancer Res.* 2004; 6(3): R170–9

Bala, M., Sawhney, R.C., et al, (eds) Sea buckthorn. A multipurpose wonder plant. Vol III: Advances in Research and Development, 2007, Dya

Publishing House, New Delhi, India, pp.254–267

Carmignani, L.O., et al, The effect of dietary soy supplementation compared to estrogen and placebo on menopausal symptoms: a randomized controlled trial. Maturitas. In Press. 2010

Ferrari, A., Soy extract phytoestrogens with high dose of isoflavones for menopausal symptoms. J. Obstet. Gynaecol. Res. 2009; Vol 35, No 6: 1083–1090

Kanadys, W.M., Leszczy ska-Gorzelak, B., Oleszczuk, J., Efficacy and safety of black cohosh (Actaea/Cimicifuga racemosa) in the treatment of vasomotor symptoms – review of clinical trials. Ginekol Pol. 2008 Apr; 79(4): 287–96

Larmo, P. S., Jarvinen, R.L., Setala, N. L., Yang, B., Viitanen, M.H., Engblom, J. R. K., Tahvonen, R.L., Kallio, H.K., Oral sea buckthorn oil attenuates tear film osmolarity and symptoms in individuals with dry eye. The Journal of Nutrition. First published ahead of print June 16, 2010 as doi: 10.3945/jn.109.118901

Liopvac, et al, Improvement of postmenopausal depressive and anxiety symptoms after treatment with isoflavones derived from red clover extracts. Maturitas 2010; 65: 258–261

Meissner, H. O., Mrozikiewicz, P., Bobkiewicz-Kozlowska, T., et al, Hormone-balancing effect of pre-gelatinized organic maca (Lepidium peruvianum Chacon) (part I) Biochemical and pharmacodynamic study on maca using clinical laboratory model on ovariectomized rats. International Journal of Biomedical Science. 2006: Vol 2, No 3. 100

Meissner, H. O., Mscisz, A., Reich-Bilinska, H., et al, Hormone-balancing effect of pre-gelatinized organic maca (Lepidium peruvianum Chacon): (II) Physiological & symptomatic responses of early-postmenopausal women to standardized doses of maca in double blind, randomized, placebo-controlled, multi-centre clinical study. International Journal of Biomedical Science. Dec 2006: Vol 2 No. 4, 360–374

Meissner, H. O., Mscisz, A., Reich-Bilinska, H., et al, Hormone-balancing effect of pre-gelatinized organic maca (Lepidium peruvianum Chacon): (III) Clinical responses of early-postmenopausal women to maca in double blind, randomized, placebo-controlled, crossover configuration, outpatient study. International Journal of Biomedical Science. Dec 2006: Vol 2 No 4, 375–394

Meissner, H. O., Reich-Bilinska, H., Mscisz, A., Kedzia, B., Therapeutic effect of Lepidium peruvianum Chacon (pre-gelatinized maca) used as a non-hormonal alternative to HRT in perimenopausal women – clinical pilot study. International Journal of Biomedical Science. 2006: Vol 2, No 2. 143

Shams, T., Setia, M.S., Hemmings, R., McCusker, J., Sewitch, M., Ciampi, A., Efficacy of black cohosh-containing preparations on menopausal symptoms: a meta-analysis. Altern Ther Health Med. 2010 Jan-Feb;16 (1): 36–44

Thompson Coon, J., Pittler, M.H., Ernst, E., The role of red clover (Trifolium pratense) isoflavones in women's reproductive health: a systematic review and meta-analysis of randomized clinical trials. Focus Altern Complement Ther. 2003; 8: 544

Van de Weijer, P.H., Barentsen, R., Isoflavones from red clover (Promensil) significantly reduce menopausal hot flush symptoms compared with placebo. Maturitas. 2002; 42(3): 187–93

Woods, R., Whitehead, M., Effects of red clover isoflavones (Promensil) versus placebo on uterine endometrium, vaginal maturation index and the uterine artery in healthy postmenopausal women. J Br Menopause Soc. 2003; SupplS2: 33

Yang, B., Lipophilic components of seeds and berries of sea buckthorn (Hippophaë rhamnoides) and physiological effects of sea buckthorn oils. 2001. Dept.of Biochemistry and Food Chem., University of Turku. ISBN951 29 2221 5

Yang, B., Bonfigli, A., et al, Effects of oral supplementation and topical application of supercritical CO_2 extracted sea buckthorn oil on skin ageing of female subjects. J. Appl. Cosmetol. 2009; 27, 1 13

Yang, B., Erkkola, R., Sea buckthorn oils, mucous membranes and Sjögren's syndrome with special reference to latest studies. In: Singh, V.; Yang, B.; Kallio, H.

Exercise and relaxation

Agıl, A., Abıke, F,. Daskapan, A., Alaca, R., Tüzün, H., Short-term exercise approaches on menopausal symptoms, psychological health, and quality of life in postmenopausal women. Obstet Gynecol Int. 2010. pii: 274261. Epub 2010 Aug 16

Di Blasio, A., Di Donato, F,. et al, Effects of the time of day of walking on dietary behaviour, body composition and aerobic fitness in postmenopausal women. J Sports Med Phys Fitness. 2010; 50(2): 196–201

Greist, J.H., Klein, M.H., Eischens, R.R., et al, Running as treatment for depression. Compr Psychiatry, 1979; 20(1): 41–54

Martin, D., Notelovitz, M., Effects of aerobic training on bone mineral density of postmenopausal women. J. Bone Miner Res. 1993; 8(8): 931–6

Nedstrand, E., Wijma, K., Wyon, Y., Hammar, M., Applied relaxation and oral estradiol treatment of vasomotor symptoms in postmenopausal women. Maturitas. 2005; 51(2): 154–62

Tüzün, S., Aktas, I., Akarirmak, U., Sipahi, S., Tüzün, F., Yoga might be an alternative training for the quality of life and balance in postmenopausal osteoporosis. Eur J Phys Rehabil Med. 2010; 46(1): 69–72

Complementary therapies

Borrelli, F., Ernst, E., Alternative and complementary therapies for the menopause. Maturitas. 2010; 66(4): 333–43. Epub 2010 Jun 30

Wyon, Y., Wijma, K., Nedstrand, E., Hammar, M. A., Comparison of acupuncture and oral estradiol treatment of vasomotor symptoms in postmenopausal women. Climacteric. 2004; 7(2): 153–64

Heart disease

Abu Mweis, S.S., Jones, P.J., Cholesterol-lowering effect of plant sterols. Curr Atheroscler Rep. 2008;10: 467–72

Li, S.H., Liu, X.X., et al, Effect of oral isoflavone supplementation on vascular endothelial function in postmenopausal women: a meta-analysis of randomized placebo-controlled trials. Am J Clin Nutr. 2009

Ortega, R.M., Palencia, A., Lopez-Sobaler, A.M., Improvement of cholesterol levels and reduction of cardiovascular risk via the consumption of phytosterols. Br J Nutr. 2006; 96: Suppl 1: S89–93

Sacks, F.M., Lichtenstein, A., Van Horn, L., Harris, W., Kris-Etherton, P., Winston, M., Soy protein, isoflavones, and cardiovascular health: an American Heart Association Science Advisory for professionals from the Nutrition Committee. *Circulation.* 2006; 113: 1034–44

Taku, K., Umegaki, K., Sato, Y., Taki, Y., Endoh, K.,Watanabe, S., Soy isoflavones lower serum total and LDL cholesterol in humans: a meta-analysis of 11 randomized controlled trials. *Am J Clin Nutr.* 2007; 85: 1148–56

Zhan, S., Ho, S.C., Meta-analysis of the effects of soy protein containing isoflavones on the lipid profile. *Am J Clin Nutr.* 2005; 81: 397–408

Osteoporosis and postmenopause

Alekel, D.L., Van Loan, M.D., Koehler, K.J., et al, The soy isoflavones for reducing bone loss (SIRBL) study: a 3-year randomized controlled trial in postmenopausal women. *Am J Clin Nutr.* 2009

Brink, E., Coxam, V., Robins, S., Wahala, K., Cassidy, A., Branca, F., Long-term consumption of isoflavone-enriched foods does not affect bone mineral density, bone metabolism, or hormonal status in early postmenopausal women: a randomized, double-blind, placebo controlled study. *Am J Clin Nutr.* 2008; 87: 761–70

Kenny, A.M., Mangano, K.M., Abourizk, R.H., et al, Soy proteins and isoflavones affect bone mineral density in older women: a randomized controlled trial. *Am J Clin Nutr.* 2009; 90: 234–42

Koh, W.P., Wu, A.H., Wang, R., et al, Gender-specific associations between soy and risk of hip fracture in the Singapore Chinese Health Study. *Am J Epidemiol.* 2009; 170: 901–9

Ma, D.F., Qin, L.Q., Wang, P.Y., Katoh, R., Soy isoflavone intake increases bone mineral density in the spine of menopausal women: meta-analysis of randomized controlled trials. *Clin Nutr.* 2008; 27: 57–64

Marini, H., Bitto, A., Altavilla, D., et al, Breast safety and efficacy of genistein aglycone for postmenopausal bone loss: a follow-up study. *J Clin Endocrinol Metab.* 2008; 93: 4787–96

Messina, M., Ho, S., Alekel, D.L., Skeletal benefits of soy isoflavones: a review of the clinical trial and epidemiologic data. *Curr Opin Clin Nutr Metab Care* 2004; 7(6):649–58

Poulsen, R.C., Kruger, M.C., Soy phytoestrogens: impact on postmenopausal bone loss and mechanisms of action. *Nutr Rev.* 2008; 66: 359–74

Vupadhyayula, P.M., Gallagher, J.C., Templin, T., Logsdon, S.M., Smith, L.M., Effects of soy protein isolate on bone mineral density and physical performance indices in postmenopausal women – a 2-year randomized, double-blind, placebo-controlled trial. *Menopause.* 2009; 16(2):320–8

Memory

Duffy, R., Wiseman, H., File, S.E., Improved cognitive function in postmenopausal women after 12 weeks of consumption of a soya extract containing isoflavones. *Pharmacol Biochem Behav.* 2003; 75(3): 721–9

Elsabagh, S., Hartley, D.E., File, S.E., Limited cognitive benefits in stage +2 postmenopausal women after six weeks of treatment with ginkgo biloba. *J Psychopharmacol.* 2005; 19(2): 173–9

File, S.E., Jarrett, N., Fluck, E., et al, Eating soya improves human memory. *Psychopharmacology.* 2001; 157(4): 430–436

Kritz-Silverstein, D., Von Muhlen, D., Barrett-Connor, E., Bressel, M.A., Isoflavones and cognitive function in older women: the soya and postmenopausal health in aging (SOPHIA) study. *Menopause.* 2003; 10(3): 196–202

Breast health

Guha, N., Kwan, M.L., Quesenberry, C.P., Jr., Weltzien, E.K., Castillo, A.L., Caan, B.J., Soy isoflavones and risk of cancer recurrence in a cohort of breast cancer survivors: the life after cancer epidemiology study. *Breast Cancer Res Treat.* 2009; 118: 395–405

Kim, H.A., Jeong, K.S., Kim, Y.K., Soy extract is more potent than genistein on tumor growth inhibition. *Anticancer Res.* 2008; 28: 2837–41

Messina, M., Hilakivi-Clarke, L., Early intake appears to be the key to the proposed protective effects of soy intake against breast cancer. *Nutr Cancer.* 2009; 61: 792–8

Messina, M., Watanabe, S., Kenneth, D. R., Setchell Report on the 8th International Symposium on the Role of Soy in Health Promotion and Chronic Disease Prevention and Treatment. *The Journal of Nutrition Supplement:* 8th International Soy Symposium: 796S–802S

Messina, M., Wood, C.E., Soy isoflavones, estrogen therapy, and breast cancer risk: analysis and commentary, *Nutrition Journal.* 2008, 7:17

Messina, M., Wu, A.H., Perspectives on the soy-breast cancer relation. *Am J Clin Nutr.* 2009; 89: 1673S–9S

Powles, T., et al, Red clover isoflavones are safe and well tolerated in women with a family history of breast cancer. *Breast Cancer Res.* 2004: 6(3): 140–142

Shu, X.O., Zheng, Y., Cai, H., et al, Soy food intake and breast cancer survival. *JAMA.* 2009; 302: 2437–43

Cancer prevention

Caan, B., Soy isoflavones and risk of cancer recurrence in a cohort of breast cancer survivors: the Life After Cancer Epidemiology study, 2009, *Breast Cancer Res Treat.*10549-009-0321-5, 2009

Guha, N., Kwan, M., Quesenberry, Jr., C., Weltzien, E., Castillo, A., Messina, M., A brief historical overview of the past two decades of soy and isoflavone research. *Journal of Nutrition.* 2010;140(7): 1350S–4S. Epub 2010 May 19

Messina, M., Hilakivi-Clarke, L., Early intake appears to be the key to the proposed protective effects of soy intake against breast cancer. *Nutr Cancer.* 2009; 61(6): 792–8

Messina, M., Watanabe, S., Setchel, K., Report on the 8th International Symposium on the Role of Soy in Health Promotion and Chronic Disease Prevention and Treatment. *Journal of Nutrition;* Supplement: 796S–802S, 2009

Messina, M., Wood, C., Soy isoflavones, estrogen therapy, and breast cancer risk: analysis and commentary, *Nutrition Journal.* 2008; 7:17

Messina, M., Wu, A.H., Perspectives on the soy-breast cancer relation. *Am J Clin Nutr.* 2009; 89(5): 1673S–1679S. Epub 2009 Apr 1

RESOURCES

For more information about the Natural Menopause Plan, please visit: www.maryonstewart.com

Maryon Stewart offers personal consultations to women all over the world. She also runs telephone workshops. For details go to: www.maryonstewart.com +44 (0)1273 609 699 enquiries@maryonstewart.com

These are some of Maryon Stewart's other books on the menopause and natural health: *Cruising Through the Menopause* Maryon Stewart (Vermilion, 2000) *The Phyto Factor* Maryon Stewart (Vermilion, 2001) *The Natural Health Bible* Maryon Stewart and Dr Alan Stewart (Vermilion, 2001)

Maryon's *Get Fit for Midlife* DVD, which is available from www.maryonstewart.com/midlifedvd, explains how the natural menopause plan helps to control symptoms of the menopause, as well as looking at how to protect your heart, bones and memory in the postmenopausal years. It also contains an exercise workout and a guided meditation. For details of the Pzizz (a power napping tool that induces a relaxed state; see page 41), go to: www.maryonstewart.com/pzizz

Stockists

Many of the supplements and other products in *The Natural Menopause Plan* are available in pharmacies, supermarkets and health food stores. You can also source specific brands online:

Note: the vitamin and mineral supplement that Maryon recommends to UK readers is Fema 45+. For US readers she recommends Gynovite. For Australian readers she recommends Blackmores Proactive Multi 50+.

For ArginMax visit:
UK www.maryonstewart.com/shop
US www.dailywellness.com
Aus www.maryonstewart.com/internationalstockists

For Arkopharma Phyto Soya products visit:
UK www.maryonstewart.com/shop
US www.maryonstewart.com/internationalstockists
Aus www.arkopharma.com.au

For Blackmores Proactive Multi 50+ (**Aus**) visit: www.blackmores.com.au

For Fema 45+ visit:
UK www.maryonstewart.com/shop

For Femenessence visit:
UK www.maryonstewart.com/shop
US/Aus www.naturalhi.com

For Omega 7 visit:
UK www.maryonstewart.com/shop
US www.aromtech.com/fi/
Aus www.bioceuticals.com.au

For Promensil visit:
UK www.maryonstewart.com/shop
US www.promensil.com/us/index.cfm
Aus www.promensil.com.au

For Regenovex visit:
UK www.maryonstewart.com/shop
US/Aus www.maryonstewart.com/internationalstockists

For Yes organic lubricant visit:
UK www.maryonstewart.com/shop
US www.naturallyforher.com
Aus www.mybodymychoice.com.au/

INDEX

ACKNOWLEDGMENTS

My first thanks must go to my patients over the last 25 years for providing me with the clinical evidence confirming the Natural Health Advisory Service Menopause Programme to be both effective and enjoyable. In particular, a big thank you goes to the patients who agreed to share their stories in this book in the unselfish hope that they could help others.

My grateful thanks must go to the other researchers around the world who have shared their work and made it possible for us to devise a workable programme.

Thanks also to Carys Glaberson, Gloria Baptist Smith and Sarah Huntley for keeping the show at the office and at home ticking over while I was otherwise occupied.

I'm enormously grateful to my family and friends for putting up with my utter preoccupation and sacrificing our shared leisure time, knowing the far-reaching health benefits the Natural Menopause Plan would offer women all around the world.